# We need to talk about this

We need to talk about this
About the new eugenics.

Copyright © 2018-2024 Angelina Souren

All rights reserved.

Essay, non-fiction, self-published.

Amazon paperback edition, 5.5" x 8.5", matte cover.

Printed on white paper in ChunkFive Roman and Bookman Old Style.

ISBN: 9781692436414

Version date: 30 July 2024

Keywords: bioethics, eugenics, assisted human reproduction, diversity, discrimination, equality, disabilities, inclusion, health, future societies, inclusivity, CRISPR, assisted reproductive technology, othering, otherization, inclusion, impairments, enhancements, ableism

**Notes**

You are not allowed to republish or translate this work or part of this work without the prior written permission from the author. That's me, Angelina Souren. Thank you for respecting the work and time that I put into this book.

I haven't referenced this book the way I would in a scientific publication because that would have made it harder to read. I have included a few references at the end of the book. Feel free to get in touch me, if you want to know more. You can contact me via angelinasouren@gmail.com. Keep in mind that my emails do not always reach me, so you may have to try a few times or contact me via a different communication channel.

# We need to talk about this

Angelina Souren

# Table of contents

| | | |
|---|---|---|
| 0. | Foreword | i |
| 1. | A provocative introduction | 1 |
| 2. | Utilitarian reasoning | 5 |
| 3. | Eugenics, old and new | 19 |
| 4. | Why we need to talk about this | 25 |
| 5. | Bias | 37 |
| 6. | Brain-based conditions | 45 |
| 7. | Lives not worth living | 63 |
| | Identity, legal persons and rights | 70 |
| 8. | A guideline for the new eugenics | 73 |
| | An exercise | 76 |
| | Implications for wrongful conception, wrongful birth and wrongful life cases | 78 |
| 9. | The bioethical imperative | 91 |
| 10. | Consequences | 97 |
| 11. | Lessons from the past and present (appendices) | 105 |
| 12. | Afterword | 129 |
| 13. | Sources of information | 133 |
| | Articles in newspapers, magazines and on blogs | 133 |
| | Books and book chapters | 148 |
| | Courses | 149 |
| | Scholarly articles and reports | 150 |
| | Videos | 158 |
| | About the author | (163) |

# Foreword

*"Life is a sexually transmitted incurable condition, fragile and tenacious at the same time."*

– Deepak Chopra

This is a book about a bioethics topic. The word "bioethics" is often interpreted as "clinical ethics" or "medical ethics", but Fritz Jahr who coined the term in 1927 saw it much broader and later came up with what he called "the bioethical imperative". I follow his, much more holistic, view of what bioethics is. It includes looking after our environment because you cannot respect other creatures and humans without also respecting their habitat.

This book was initially inspired by Michael Sandel and Glenn Cohen and I gratefully tip my cap at them, as well as at the always so amicable Hank Greely and Brian Earp. Writing this book was also sparked by real-life people around me in Britain as well as by people who were or became part of my life in the past, such as friends and family.

While I do not wish to give off the impression that I am ignoring the contributions of Marianne K., Astrid F., Jetty A., Paul S. and many others, I owe a great deal to three women scientists who have played a big role in my life, namely Hélène van Pinxteren, Kine Sittig and Julie Siler.

In March 2017, when I was still in the middle of writing the first edition of this book, expert Wendy Savage (who is a gynecologist as well as a professor at Cambridge University in Britain) allegedly stated in an interview with the Daily Mail that a pregnant woman should always be told the sex of the fetus and should be allowed to abort the fetus if she does not like the baby's sex. That highlights how necessary it is to have these discussions. For starters, gender is not a binary switch, but on top of that, a practice as allegedly proposed by Savage (making sex selection permissible) would also clear the road for deselecting a fetus for just about any discriminatory reason. It turns babies into products, like pink and pastel-blue handbags. Isn't this what the term "designer babies" is all about?

Besides having changed the gender compositions of some populations, we have also already changed the populations of countries like Iceland, Denmark and the U.S. by eradicating children with Down syndrome. At the same time, we are seeing a surprising trend of emancipation for people with Down. Allow someone to flourish boundlessly and you may be astonished by what he or she turns out to be capable of. ("Treat people as if they were what they should be, and you help them become what they are capable of becoming," Goethe is supposed to have said or, more likely, written a long time ago.) Hold people back, lock them away into institutions, where you sometimes even chain them to walls or beds, and you condemn them to a life of limitations. The brain craves input. The brain craves connection. Besides, we've also seen this same evolution happen for women to some degree. Our brains too were supposed to be unsuitable for academic endeavors. It was said to hamper our fertility and mess with our reproductive organs.

The previous two editions were still quite clumsily written here and there and I hope that I didn't step on too many toes. Partly, they were an exercise in logical reasoning – doodles – to arrive at various definitions, for example of what "a life not worth living" might be, and to come up with a guideline that I know is never going to be used in practice. (That's still true of this edition too.)

Then a Chinese scientist called He Jiankui made the spotlights because he'd broken all the rules by creating real-life CRISPR'd babies. On 11 February 2023, Dr He attended his first public event since his release, namely the conference "Looking Back into the Future: CRISPR and Social Values" organized by Dr Joy Zhang at the University of Kent. What struck me during that meeting was not so much He's perceived arrogance or deception, but the attitude of many scientists, particularly those in very early stages of their careers. I later also saw that reflected at two meetings that I attended in the Netherlands. The idea of pondering the potential consequences of their research does not seem to occur to many scientists. In addition, they often see ethics committees as no more than groups of pesky people who want them to tick boxes. This worries me, but I understand it. I too used to be very enthusiastic about all science, particularly if it concerned my own favorite areas. I am sure that I never paid any thoughts to possible consequences of mining operations when I was much younger, not just in terms of pollution but

# Foreword

also with regard to impact on communities and wildlife. This is probably a point at which I should interject that I went to university relatively late; the issue is not age-related but experience-related.

I mustn't forget to mention that CRISPR has many versions and that a very important distinction is that between germline editing in which traits are altered and passed on to offspring and editing that only affects one individual. The new eugenics is very rapidly becoming a reality, however. It means that we need to have a discussion about the degree to which ableism or mainstreamism plays a role in our decisionmaking and how we are treating each other at the moment. We mustn't overlook the role of how we are dealing with the wide range in human diversity in society right now. There is still so much room for progress and improvement in that area and it is intimately connected with the discussion about the use of techniques like CRISPR in germline editing. That is what this book is about.

I could have called this book "The honey mustard chicken society" after the title of a video made by a chronically ill woman who is preparing honey mustard chicken. The woman in question is genetically different from mainstream people. The main differences are a gene mutation and a mitochondrial condition. This was diagnosed when she was about 15 years old. It has many practical consequences including the fact she can't just eat anything she wants. That led to her video about her honey mustard chicken meal.

That title would have captured the duality of the questions surrounding the new eugenics. You could say that the central question in this book is whether non-mainstream people, like the woman in that video, should get to eat their honey mustard chicken or not. Should we weed them out from the human species as unwanted or undesirable or to spare them pain and discomfort? This may sound trivial but it's not. When Glenn Cohen talks about intentional diminishment with regard to genetically deaf parents who want genetically deaf children, isn't that ableism? This is the big issue. Why is it objectionable to create genetically deaf children to allow them to experience the richness of deaf culture and make them feel included in their family and community but should it be okay to do the reverse? There is also the chicken. The chicken has rights too. Shouldn't the chicken too get to live her life freely? How can a society claim to be advanced if it still depends on the ruthless exploitation of other species for its food supply? Shouldn't we simply be able to produce clean, tasty, cruelty-free food instead? How can we reconcile some of the conflicting interests that come to the fore in these discussions?

This is why we need to talk about what kind of society we want our grandchildren to live in and we need to do this before we set ourselves on a course that may be hard to change later. Do we want a world that forces people to be a certain way, such as in the film "The Stepford Wives"? Do we want a society that divides people into separate superior and inferior classes such as in the film "Gattaca" and in the novel "The Ultimate Brainchild"? Or do we prefer one that embraces all diversity, in principle, and sees the good in the "bad". It might be better to cherish a society that accepts that good and bad are not separable but relative and hence quite normal. Most diversity comes with unique abilities and vital viewpoints that we might lose if we start fixing things that do not need to be fixed. Autism is not a mental illness and does not compare at all to schizophrenia, for example, but both are often seen as similar. That is probably like saying that color-blindness is comparable to diabetes.

I think that, within the context of assisted human reproduction (the new eugenics), we should primarily focus on using these technologies to enable life, for now. We don't have enough knowledge yet to allow it to be taken forward freely. Several other developments still need to run their course and will address some of the questions that the new eugenics could be trying to address. Focusing the new eugenics on enabling life, for now, makes it much easier to come up with a logical universal guideline that can be applied and can then be extended stepwise. By "enabling life" I mean "enabling embryos to develop into adults". I will come back to this when I explain my definition of "a life not worth living".

This also means that mitochondrial replacement therapy (MRT) should be allowed, as is already the case in several countries. MRT is about enabling life and about curing. It is not an expression of a preference for one child over another.

My background is in science and technology, not in bioethics, and there are a million things that I don't know. Who am I to write a book like this? I find it hard to stay silent in a world in which so many people seem focused on getting the latest iPhone, don't talk with the neighbors because the neighbors are probably not "one of us" or look the other way and stay silent when they know they should speak up. The way I see it, if you are born with a lot of strength, in any area, some of that

# Foreword

endowment is given to you for the specific purpose of looking out for and standing up for others who may be less able to do that.

After He Jiankui was released from prison in China and the first CRISPR treatments such as Casgevy and Lyfgenia started receiving approval in countries like the UK and the US, it was time to tweak the book slightly and weed out any remaining typos. I also needed to define its audience more clearly. This is not quite a book for lay people, but it is suitable for any researchers. That I don't have a background in CRISPR research will become clear soon enough for anyone who is familiar with it. The purpose of this book wasn't to start talking about off-target effects or discuss that making someone immune to HIV, the way He Jiankui did with Nana and Lulu and possibly a third baby, may make them vulnerable to other conditions. The contents of some of the chapters have barely changed since the first edition, which I published in 2017.

The quotations at the start of the chapters are only meant as inspiration. It does not matter that much who said what. What matters is that someone did and that you should consume that idea and see what you can do with it. The flaws in this book are all mine. If you spot any errors or typos in the book, feel free to let me know (angelinasouren@gmail.com). In this digital age, it is usually very easy for me to remedy imperfections, allowing me to provide later readers with a slightly more pleasant experience, even though I no longer have the original files. I thank you in advance!

# 1. A provocative introduction

*"Britain now finds itself at the forefront of the new eugenics."*

– Fraser Nelson, The Spectator, April 2016

Let's carry out a thought experiment. Imagine a western country that is the most openly misogynistic country in the world. (The word "misogyny" means "hostility and hate toward women", which is what sexism often boils down to in practice.) If you're a fetus in that western country, you currently have a greater-than-30% chance of being born into poverty and the level of poverty in that country is often pretty bad. No chickenshit. Significant deep poverty. Dickensian poverty.

Every winter, tens of thousands of people die in that country because they can't afford to heat their homes properly. If you're one of those 30 or 40% of its poor children, your health and learning abilities are likely to suffer as a result of the poverty you grow up in, your lifespan will probably be shorter, and both the level and the quality of the education you receive is bound to be lower. You are also more likely to become homeless as the financial support for young people in this country is highly limited and flawed, and most wages are low.

Let's assume that this western country is part of the EU. The country's inequality is so immense that on its own, it drags down socioeconomic (in)equality for the entire EU. So it pulls down the combined value for the other 27 countries. Again, no chickenshit. In addition, there is a lot of xenophobia including colonialism, gerontophobia and general intolerance and distrust, not just with regard to persons from other countries – this is often called "insularity" – but also within the country itself, among its own citizens. Also, research has revealed that this country's citizens are also the loneliest people in the EU, and possibly of the entire world.

The level of education among the population in this country isn't necessarily very high, although it has a handful of elitist universities that consider themselves important and beat themselves on the chest, while more and more of the country's students prefer to do their degrees in the U.S. Many Chinese high-school students perform better than that country's best high-school students and those Chinese students also have a better command of that western country's language.

The country's people are far from stupid, however. In fact, most are pretty clever. They wouldn't survive otherwise. There is an understandably high level of alcohol abuse, which constitutes a major drain on the country's health system. There is also, not so surprising, a significant level of crime and a high level of various forms of injustice (including several instances of mass child sex abuse of a nature that other countries don't appear to have).

The level of knowledge and training has been gradually sliding over the past 100 years or so, so that this country now requires foreigners to help keep its power plants and hospitals running.

As a country, it doesn't cooperate particularly well with other countries. The nation's leaders are often perceived as obnoxious or immature by the leaders of many other nations. Its national manner of thinking is generally described as "muddled", also by people from that country who have extensive international experience, such as major diplomats. These diplomats sometimes even quit when they become too frustrated, too fed up with having to deal with too much childish, muddled and dishonest stuff from their own government.

The country also likes to wage wars. It has managed to have one of the longest armed conflicts in the history of humanity, fought a war against Argentina in which a little over 900 people were killed just a few decades ago and has announced that it won't hesitate to begin a war against Spain either.

Now, if NATO and the UN were to get together, and decided to bomb this country to smithereens and turn it into a nature reserve, everyone would benefit. Nobody would suffer. Except maybe that country's representatives in NATO and the UN, but that's all. If those few folks were sent home in advance, they'd never even realize what was happening so that, surely, would be the humane thing to do. The country's inhabitants would cease to suffer – they would be put out of their misery – and prevention of harm is a good thing, of course. Everyone else would clearly benefit as well because they would no longer have to endure the negative effects of this country's bad habits and attitudes. Spain could sleep easier. On top of that, everyone would gain a wonderful nature reserve.

# A provocative introduction

No problem, right?

(I hope you are fuming now.)

If this thought experiment about eliminating a country based on the argument that its destruction would increase the good in the world and decrease harm makes you feel uneasy, upset or angry, then consider that elimination of groups of humans takes place all the time. The composition of countries' populations and thus the world's population is changing as a result.

Non-mainstream people are often considered less desirable or assumed to be miserable. This can include "disabled" people but also people who are not financially wealthy, who have a different lifestyle or who speak a dialect. People who are different are not only sometimes banned from shops and towns, or schools. They are often also banned from life, as a matter of course. This happens when future parents select or de-select a certain type of offspring. Sometimes the law of their country tells them to do that. At other times, medical professionals tell them to choose science over nature or make an informed decision.

How do you think the people feel whose kind is being eradicated? How happy do you think they are about being considered undesirable? Not cool or sexy enough? How do you think they feel about their elimination supposedly being beneficial for everyone else?

I am referring to the new eugenics, the practice of creating designer babies at the expense of less desirable babies. This is not a new thing. It's been happening for a while. A designer baby is any kind of baby that is considered more desirable than another kind of viable baby. It's like only choosing handbags by Debenhams and rejecting handbags by Marks & Spencer. Isn't it ironic that over the course of the various editions of this book, my beloved Debenhams has ceased to exist? That's exactly what I mean when I ask for caution. Circumstances can change in unexpected ways.

**We need** to talk about this

## 2. Utilitarian reasoning

*"There is only one success: to be able to live your life in your own way."*

– Christopher Morley

The thought experiment in Chapter 1, about the country of which the annihilation supposedly would benefit everyone, hence justifying the country's destruction, is an example of utilitarian reasoning.

Although the word "utilitarian" is often used as almost synonymous with "spartan" these days, that is not at all what I am referring to when I use the terms "utilitarian" and "utilitarianism". Instead, I have a way of thinking, a philosophy, in mind, or more precisely, the way this philosophy is often applied in practice. Within the context of utilitarianism, the word "utility" stands for something close to "pleasure" or "usefulness".

Utilitarianism was a school of thought that had a huge impact on 19th-century Britain, where it sprung up and blossomed. It still exercises a strong influence. Utilitarianism appears to go a long way toward explaining why we don't accept ourselves and each other the way we are, and why we have so much inequality and bias in British society. Could it also have a lot to do with why Britain has this strange hierarchical class system that divides people into undeserving, lower types of people and entitled, higher types of humans?

The idea behind utilitarianism as a school of thought was that the right thing to do was that which produced the greatest amount of good for the greatest number of people. A simple example of what it can mean in practice would probably be that if you are stuck in an elevator for a long time, say, after an earthquake, it would be okay to start eating one of the people in the elevator as that person's demise might ensure the survival of the others who are stuck on the elevator. Who would you be willing to kill and eat, and why would you pick that specific person?

Unfortunately, utilitarian reasoning makes it possible to define for yourself what "good" is and hence claim that you are justified to do something intrinsically bad (harmful to someone else) because it benefits you. It can include attaching a higher value to certain people to arrive at a greater amount of good that would be accomplished for them. You could probably say that what happened in Nazi Germany was an example of utilitarian reasoning. Nazi-style eugenics even bears some resemblance to specific ideas that the founders of utilitarianism entertained.

I want to emphasize, however, that this discussion is not about what utilitarianism should be or how it was intended. It is about its actual application. You can use a fishing pole to catch fish and you can use it to grab someone else's bucket of fish. You might even be able to hit someone over the head with the heavy end of a fishing pole and then take that person's catch. It's not the fishing pole's fault. It can be used for good and it can be used for bad. Most people use it for good. The same holds for water. YouTube has plenty of videos showing people who give water to parched wildlife, but water is also part of a torture method used at Guantánamo Bay (the United States military prison on Cuba). It is not the water's fault.

When you start talking about guns, something shifts because it is harder to do any kind of good with a gun. Utilitarianism is somewhere in between. It is not an innocent kind of reasoning. It is not intrinsically neutral but intrinsically biased, just like a gun is intrinsically positively biased toward the person holding the gun. A gun represents power and so does utilitarian reasoning; they both seem to create as well as support a power imbalance.

This has allowed utilitarianism to result in callous excesses and the abandonment of morality or justice to make way for cold-hearted calculations. The idea of "what is the morally, ethically right thing to do" is sometimes sacrificed in favor of "what is the cheapest thing to do" or simply "what do I like best" in utilitarian reasoning.

I found out about utilitarianism after I relocated to Britain, and I often found myself shocked by the displays of callousness around me. I had never encountered anything like it before and I wondered where it came from.

I also saw a lot of unhappy people, more than I'd ever encountered elsewhere. One of the first clues as to what was going on came when I spotted a job advert in a window one day, for a store manager, listing a surprisingly low salary. As I was self-employed and working with clients

## Utilitarian reasoning 7

in other countries, I had not caught on yet at that point that so many salaries in the U.K. were much lower than in my home country.

I spoke with one landlord who considered it not sad but a great inconvenience to himself that one of his tenants had tried to commit suicide. It made him angry. He considered such tenants bad tenants. This also went for tenants who called him if the heating or the washing machine provided by him was not working. On one occasion, he confided in me that he felt that people who aren't educated were objectionable to him. I was so shocked that I was unable to reply at the time. The same person also advises the courts in child custody cases. How on earth can he keep his personal bias out of the advice he offers the courts?

Maybe surprisingly, he is actually a good man. He is not a bad person at all, not at all. So how could a person like that say such horrible cruel things? Maybe Aldous Huxley answered that in Brave New World: "One believes things because one has been conditioned to believe them."

Another landlord I talked with told me how he had tricked an older lady with beginning Alzheimer's disease out of her home and got her to move into a bigger flat, with more rooms than she was able to use. He also said to me about a new building he was constructing that it was "only for tenants, so it does not have to be very good".

Thankfully, there are still plenty of kind and compassionate people in Britain, despite that trend of unfettered greed at the expense of everything and everyone else. Appalled, I have watched all sorts of people make fun of and seemingly enjoy other people's hardships in Britain, though. Iain Duncan Smith (or "IDS") comes to mind as an example.

There seems to be a general lack of conscience and accountability in the country, certainly also on the side of the government and among politicians, particularly on the side of the Conservatives but also on the side of what used to be called UKIP but is called the Brexit Party at the time of writing (and Labour and the LibDems may not be as far behind as they think they are). Also in everyday life, there is an acceptance of callousness and of lying that I had not witnessed before. No, it does not compare at all to what Donald Trump has been doing, because when he lies, he believes that he is telling the truth. (He's not trying to fool you. He's trying to reassure himself.) It is not the kind of "lying" that comes from genuinely perceiving a different truth either (although that, too, occurs a lot among Conservatives, I must say, because they live in a bubble or, as one of their greatest local fans would call it, "they are blinkered").

Where did all of this come from, I wondered? I set out to understand. I started reading books about Britain's history. I sometimes asked people questions, such as why they were much more sociable than others around them. Victorianism (Puritanism) provided half of the answer to explain the mystery that the U.K. presented to me, but something was still missing. Eventually, I stumbled upon utilitarianism and saw that this was the missing information that I had been looking for.

Two privileged white men drove utilitarianism, Jeremy Bentham (1748-1832) who invented it and his disciple John Stuart Mill (1806-1873) who carried it forward. They did not set out to harm anyone, but their experience of the world appears to have been very limited. (I'll come back to that.)

Bentham was ahead of his time, surely, in his endeavors to make homosexuality a private matter instead of a crime. Unfortunately, he apparently overlooked that the way he phrased his ideas might also clear the way for considering child sex abuse merely a private matter.

Mill pushed feminism because he noticed the extent to which society and its customs had held back his wife. It is interesting that he appears to have used the phrase "social disability" to describe that phenomenon. It is interesting because it hints at the notion that many "disabilities" are not problematic by themselves but because of hindrances that society inadvertently creates for people who do not match the traditional ideal of the wealthy white male Olympian sports hero.

Utilitarianism had a massive impact on British society because Bentham and Mill weren't academics tucked away behind desks in ivory towers. Bentham was a legal reformer and Mill was a civil servant and a national politician (Member of Parliament, or MP), a public figure. Notably many of Mill's general ideas were well known among the working class.

While utilitarianism isn't the overall encouragement of spartan conditions but the application of calculations in decision-making and policy development, Bentham certainly envisaged spartan conditions for specific groups of people.

Bentham proposed to round up the beggars because their visible presence decreased the happiness of the more fortunate, according to him. He wanted them in workhouses, in an order that, also according to him, would reduce unhappiness. He also wanted the deaf and dumb "next to raving lunatics, or persons of profligate conversation", aged women next to "prostitutes and loose women", and the blind next to the "shockingly deformed".

This is the opposite of accepting human diversity. This is a way of classifying humans, of declaring some humans as less worthy, as less valuable. This constitutes avoidance of anyone who is non-mainstream. This declares people who aren't the traditional sports hero type lesser beings. It also ignores and insults their intelligence.

Bentham could just as easily have reasoned that the sight of the wealthy, average-bodied and healthy caused the beggars, deaf and dumb and blind discomfort and hurt. He could have said that it was the others' duty to increase the happiness of those whose visible presence, he thought, was offensive. He could have decided that this meant that the well-to-do had to adopt a beggar in their household or that intellectuals had to take people who were less intelligent under their wing and that those with 20/20 vision should take a blind person by the arm. But he didn't.

Instead of looking to maximize happiness, he focused on reducing unhappiness in his own group of people. It reflected his own discomfort, the unease he must have felt when he saw people who were in very different circumstances. "Oh, my god, that could have been me, that beggar there on the corner. I don't want to be confronted with that. Off to the workhouse you go." We currently see this approach a lot in the U.K. Towns criminalize homelessness, while economic homelessness continues to skyrocket. Many people, also those in work, frequently find themselves faced with the choice "do I top up my prepaid electricity, do I buy food or do I set something aside for the rent while the electricity goes off and I have nothing to eat?" Homeless people are forcibly removed from underpasses and doorways. Poor families sometimes get relocated across distances of hundreds of kilometers, away from friends and family. New residential buildings sometimes have a door at the back to be used by their poor residents; flats for poor people are often included in buildings that predominantly house the rich because it can result in planning permission.

Bentham's disciple John Stuart Mill pushed utilitarianism further into inequality by distinguishing between lower and higher pleasures. Biological pleasures, such as the pleasure derived from enjoying a sheer necessity – food – or from enjoying sex were lower pleasures, in his view. Mill considered reading Shakespeare a higher pleasure. You could just as easily declare food a higher pleasure, however, as Shakespeare and chess are no good and not enjoyable to anyone who has not eaten any food in a long time.

Yet even today, many still consider it better to read Shakespeare or play chess than to watch Grey's Anatomy, play football or enjoy the Simpsons, even though in practice, most people like the Simpsons more and therefore derive more pleasure from it, as political philosopher Michael Sandel has often pointed out in his classes at Harvard Law School and in his books. Can't we just say that they're both equally valuable and be done with it? There is nothing wrong with playing chess and there is nothing wrong with playing football.

If you use utilitarian reasoning, you can also see a string necklace of genuine pearls as more useful to a rich socialite than to the average Goth, even though the Goth might sell the necklace and get a year's worth of food out of it as the Goth's pleasure would rank lower than the socialite's pleasure because the Goth's pleasure would be seen as a lower pleasure. It might even justify stealing the pearls from the Goth to give them to the socialite.

Does all of this also help explain why some people perceive humans with lower IQs as less valuable? Bioethicist Julian Savulescu has argued that people with average IQs lack the ability to enjoy intellectual activities and that by "enhancing" the human race so that these so-called higher pleasures would become available to everyone, we would do ourselves a favor and increase our collective joy. But who determines what the greater joy is? Just like beauty is in the eye of the beholder, so is pleasure.

A high IQ provides no protection against poverty or illness, or even against car accidents or child abuse and a high IQ does not guarantee financial success either. "If you're so smart, why aren't you rich?" was the heading for an article in MIT's Technology Review in November 2019. Financial success or success in business is mostly due to chance, it turns out.

By the way, France had briefly seen something similar to utilitarianism

## Utilitarian reasoning 11

before Bentham came along. It was proposed by Claude-Adrien Helvétius in the 18th century. In the country that now has "brotherhood, equality and freedom" as its national motto, these ideas were condemned so strongly – partly even banned – that they soon disappeared again.

The division in higher and lower pleasures was mainly Mill's response to criticisms on Bentham's utilitarianism. In Britain, many saw Bentham's utilitarianism as a doctrine for swine (the mere chasing of pleasures), to which Mill retorted that it was better to have an unhappy human than a happy pig, and so he came up with the division into lower and higher pleasures. He clearly saw no point in trying to make a pig happy as that would only result in "lower" pleasures, according to him.

Isn't this also what we saw in Britain when its Tory governments imposed austerity measure after austerity measure primarily on those who would be hardest hit by these measures, not caring how many lives were lost as a result, even laughing about it out loud when suicides were mentioned in Parliament? (Tories are Conservatives on the far right, with extreme, feudal views.) Isn't that also utilitarian reasoning when many U.K. politicians consider it desirable to have millions and millions of Brits – including children and chronically ill people – live in extended deep poverty and consider it fine to lie to the British public about anything as long as it will get them (re)elected? Austerity became an even crazier story when it turned out that the U.K. government had hundreds of billions available to spend on everything to do with Brexit, even when it was not sure yet whether Brexit would go ahead.

The 19th century heavily stamped its mark on Britain and many people in Britain still hanker after those days. Many have also said this within the context of Brexit, as surprising as it may sound. We're well into the 21st century and no other country appears to display this kind of hang-up, although you sometimes see something similar among certain extremists who still yearn for the Ottoman Empire of the past. At the same time, there is also a rebellion in British society against many of those 19th-century values, sometimes also leading to excesses.

Of John Stuart Mill, we know that he looked down on the British working class. He considered them nothing but liars.

Mill put great emphasis on intellectual pleasures. How could he not? He was home-schooled and his father started him on reading classical Greek at age 3. He began learning Latin soon after and read Homer in the original Latin at age 7 or thereabouts. I think it is fair to say that Mill's views on life were probably somewhat distorted. Wouldn't he in fact have declared a large part of his own life a failure or a life of cultural poverty if he had openly placed at least as much value on other types of pleasure than the ones he had indulged in?

His mentor Bentham went to Oxford University at age 12, where he studied law. As he was well to do, he did not need a job and was free to pursue his own pleasures. He was one of the founders of what later became University College London. He also founded a utilitarian newspaper called the Westminster Review. I think that we can surely also say of Bentham that he wrote from the exclusive perspective of a privileged man. As he never required any form of employment, he can't have experienced what it is like to be without a limitless supply of safety and security or to be in desperate need of food and shelter.

In spite of that, Bentham did feel that the principle of right and wrong was often no more than an expression of personal likes and dislikes. Legislation should, therefore, be based on calculations, and on maximizing happiness, he said. However, in utilitarianism, happiness is not defined by the person experiencing happiness or unhappiness, but by the person who has the upper hand.

Bentham wasn't a strong believer in individual rights, even though he felt that everyone should at least have the right to be protected from physical harm. Keep this in mind, for example, for when you get to the Ford Pinto example.

Bentham seemed to believe that violations of rights were linked to people's abilities, in the sense that less "able" people would not notice certain things done to them or happening around them, making the offenses less serious or maybe even permissible in those cases. It is important to note this. Is it acceptable for a shopkeeper to shortchange someone with an IQ of 85 and, for instance, sell him or her a phone that won't work or to give a blind person a torn and dirty dress because that person might not notice it?

(This is why we now have universally declared human rights. They were put in place after the atrocities that happened in Nazi Germany when many people were declared undesirable and disposable merely because they were not the blond, blue-eyed sports hero type. Britain was one of the architects of these universally declared human rights, even though the Tories have been ridiculing them as an evil EU invention that forces Britain to let terrorists into the country and provide prisoners with their daily dose of pornography.)

While Mill was not keen on the British working class, he wasn't very fond of the British in general either. He considered them "parochial" and took pride in being able to read and communicate in French. Mill first visited France at the age of 14 and reported that he enjoyed the "free and genial atmosphere of Continental life" very much. What would have happened to that if France had not rejected the ideas of Helvétius? Mill also noticed that the French didn't suppress their feelings, whereas 19th-century Britons did. Both Mill and his father didn't know what to do with emotions. Again, is it any wonder that the younger Mill placed so much emphasis on intellectual pleasures?

What Mill had not foreseen, it seems, is that this suppression or dismissal of feelings combined with utilitarian calculations could result in an occasionally somewhat psychopathic application of utilitarianism, the sweeping aside of moral principles to make way for (financial) cost-benefit analyses. As I've already mentioned, the problem with the utilitarian approach is that it can too easily be twisted to suit one's personal aims.

Unintentionally, Bentham and Mill had created a theoretical instrument that allowed people to do harm and explain it away, more or less according to the following reasoning.

1. All my actions are allowed unless they cause harm (Mill in On Liberty).

2. If my actions cause harm, then a simple calculation usually suffices to justify my actions anyway (Bentham and Mill).

3. If my calculation doesn't seem to add up in my favor, then I can assign higher values to some effects of my actions relative to other effects, for example by declaring myself more important than someone else, and then I can still get away with doing harm because it allows me to claim that I still do more good than harm (Mill, in Utilitarianism). It's a matter of weighting the accomplished pleasure, gains or happiness in order to be able to dismiss someone else's discomfort, loss or pain.

Thus, utilitarianism fosters inequality.

By the way, I sometimes wonder if utilitarianism also resulted in the view that seems to be held in some circles that a person is naive or unsophisticated if he or she objects to a certain course of action because he or she considers it morally wrong (even though someone else stands to gain a lot of money or power from it).

Here are some examples of how utilitarian reasoning can work out in practice.

- If 10 robbers kill one rich person to steal that person's gemstones, you can say that more people will benefit from the theft of the gemstones and that it outweighs the harm done by killing the rich person. But if one poor person steals the gemstones, then you can say that the rich person loses more than the poor person gains because the poor ("inferior") person is assessed as not able to appreciate the monetary or aesthetic value of the gemstones, hence unable to derive any pleasure from them. (This is an example I've made up.)

- When the Ford Motor Company in the United States refused a recall of its Pinto model, it reasoned that remedying the problem with the Pinto would be more expensive than paying out damages for the (apparently inferior) people who were killed or injured as a result of Pintos bursting into flames. The pleasure for the company was greater if it simply paid out for the victims than if it prevented their deaths and injuries. (This example comes from Michael Sandel's publication "Justice – What's the right thing to do".)

- When British politician Iain Duncan Smith openly doubled over with laughter in a televised session of Parliament when another politician was in the middle of explaining the plight of poor ("inferior") people with handicaps and chronic illnesses ("inferior"), and mentioned that deaths had occurred as a result of harsh measures implemented by that specific politician, that laughing politician was applying his own utilitarian views. Cutting financial support for the country's poorest and most vulnerable made it possible for him to balance the country's books at the expense of the people whose income got cut and still have more than enough left in the country's coffers to use for purely political purposes. Utilitarian reasoning could even

## Utilitarian reasoning 15

see those deaths as positive as those people now no longer needed to be supported, which could easily be put in terms of achieving greater overall happiness. In the period between the 2016 Brexit referendum and the December 2019 election, huge amounts of money still turned out to be available that dwarfed the peddled financial benefits of Brexit and those benefits – the so-called Brexit dividend – had turned out to be a complete lie. (This is an example from real life.)

- When governments deliberately keep a large section of the population disproportionately poor, enabling such governments to realize major budget cuts in times of economic crisis such as the one that precipitated around 2008 as a result of bankers' misconduct, you also have utilitarianism in action. Such governments treat the poor like cattle that they sell off to be slaughtered or buy to be fed depending on the county's financial situation. It is easy to see this as the result of a simple utilitarian financial cost-benefit analysis. If you keep a large group of people disproportionately poor and relatively uneducated, at all times, then it becomes much harder for them to fight back against anything you do to them and it also becomes near-impossible for them to work their way out of poverty. It means that you can use them as a tool, as a commodity. Like cattle. This was the situation that Iain Duncan Smith made use of. If this situation had not already existed, cuts would not have had such dramatic consequences for so many. (This is an example from real life.)

- When a group of people zips around through the streets, high on excitement, because someone has just jumped off a bridge to commit suicide, that's utilitarianism in action. The pleasure experienced by the people excited by the suicide outweighs the lack of pleasure experienced by the person who committed suicide. It gets even worse – or better; if you happen to use a utilitarian point of view – when a group of people egg someone on to jump off a building. (These too are real-life examples.)

- When police officers sided with youngsters who threw eggs and stones at the house of a Frenchwoman in Devon, was that based on a utilitarian calculation? Was the "fun" that was enjoyed by the British youngsters more important than the discomfort, anger and fear experienced by the Frenchwoman? (This is an example from real life.)

- Landlords or builders who openly state that a new building is only for tenants, and therefore doesn't have to be very good or who use unsuitable materials when those materials are cheaper also practice utilitarianism. They consider lowering their expenses the greater good over raising the comfort of tenants or even lowering the tenants' costs of living (which would benefit these landlords too, but they appear to be blind to that). (These are examples from real life.)

- Convicting a person who is known to be innocent in order to pacify a larger group of people who genuinely believe that this person is guilty, that's utilitarianism. (This example is often mentioned in explanations of utilitarianism.) By the way, in Britain, there is no compensation for such wrongly convicted and imprisoned people, and even people entitled to compensation, such as the victims of the Windrush scandal or disabled people who experienced illegal cuts to their financial support, often wait many years to receive that compensation.

- The casual acceptance of mass child sex abuse too can be seen as a form of utilitarianism. How important is the misery of a few children when compared against the perverse pleasures experienced by a large number of children's home employees or by a TV personality? This type of utilitarian attitude allows anyone to brush the children's interests aside as of insufficient significance. (This is an example from real life.)

- When shop staff deliberately takes advantage of persons they consider mentally (or physically) inferior, that's utilitarianism. (This is an example from real life.)

- When there is a greater chance that a poor ("inferior") person who stole a sandwich and was identified on CCTV is arrested and prosecuted than someone who commits far more serious crimes, could that too be an expression of utilitarianism? (This is an example from real life.)

- Constant lying can easily be seen as a form of utilitarianism as well. The gains you accomplish by the lying outweigh the harm done to the people you lie to, says the utilitarian calculation. (This is a general observation.)

- In London, some buildings have (back) entrances for the poor and (front) entrances for the wealthy. (Allowing less well-off tenants in their buildings can help developers get planning permission.) I hear the echo of Bentham's teachings in this, too, in the idea that the rich might be offended (harmed) by seeing the less well-off tenants using the same entrance. In New York, a block was found to have been approved with a so-called poor door at about the same time as this phenomenon came to light in London. There, it caused a roar. Mayor Bill De Blasio said that he would take action to prevent this from happening in the future. By contrast, poor doors were already becoming standard practice in London by then.

- When Britain's leaders fed the voters lies, for example about the ability of EU citizens to claim benefits as soon as they set foot in the country (which they couldn't), they were also applying utilitarianism. This kind of lie brought these politicians votes (on false grounds) and helped foster more negativity toward foreigners. When that results in less interaction with those foreigners, there is also a smaller chance for Brits to discover the truth.

- In 2006, Prime Minister Tony Blair argued in a BBC interview that children should be taken away from certain parents, even before birth, even if for no other reason than that those children supposedly would "only grow up to become hooligans" and that this would cost society too much money later. This too is sheer utilitarianism. It declares some parents' happiness less valuable because of their socioeconomic status. (In the distant future, society may decide to make parenting a profession and require training and licenses before parents are allowed to have children, but that is a far cry from taking children away from their parents in the present situation, just because the parents are of a certain class.) Sadly, Blair managed to turn this into law right before the end of his final term.

Doesn't particularly the kind of thinking shown in the latter example – social engineering – make the step to mandatory eugenics uncomfortably small? Isn't Tony Blair's approach very similar to what several Tory politicians have been saying, namely that the poor shouldn't be allowed to reproduce? There is little room for respect for individual humans who are perceived as "inferior" or "diminished" in these skewed expressions of utilitarianism.

"Britain now finds itself at the forefront of the new eugenics", wrote Fraser Nelson in British magazine The Spectator in April 2016. He pointed out that Britain had also laid the foundation for old-style eugenics. That too emerged in the 19th century, along with Victorianism and utilitarianism. Is their co-incidence a mere coincidence?

## 3. Eugenics, old and new

*"The only way of cutting off the constant stream of idiots and imbeciles and feeble-minded persons who help to fill our prisons and workhouses, reformatories, and asylums is to prevent those who are known to be mentally defective from producing offspring. Undoubtedly the best way of doing this is to place these defectives under control. Even if this were a hardship to the individual it would be necessary for the sake of protecting the race."*

– The Spectator, 25 May 1912


*"My life would be rather simple if people would consider me as a person rather than a thing to eradicate."*

– Nicolas Joncour, 2016


Eugenics is the deliberate process of "improving" the human species. It isn't a new invention, of course. Most people probably associate the term "eugenics" with the excesses that happened in Germany barely a lifetime ago during the Second World War. Old-style eugenics began in Britain, however, not in Germany. The Victorian-era ideas of Francis Galton were adopted by the United States, from where they provided the inspiration for Nazi Germany's practices. Old-style eugenics is still taking place in the world today, now reinforced by the new eugenics (consumer eugenics). Chapter 11 contains illustrative examples harvested mostly from the internet.

The old and the new eugenics overlap, of course. The new eugenics – the selection and de-selection of embryos and fetuses on the basis of properties, and the addition, alteration or elimination of genes or gene combinations in embryos and fetuses – more or less began with chorionic villus sampling (CVS) and amniocentesis. It enabled us to abort certain fetuses if they were diagnosed with certain conditions.

Then we started buying and selecting donor eggs and donor sperm, ticking off boxes with properties that we were looking for. How much freedom you have in these matters still depends on in which country you shop for these services, though.

Since 1989, we've been carrying out pre-implantation genetic diagnosis (PGD), also known as pre-implantation genetic screening (PGS), on the pre-embryos created during in-vitro fertilization (IVF). IVF is a rapidly growing market.

Old-style eugenics was conducted by nations and states.

In the new-style eugenics, parents are supposedly free to choose and not exposed to undue influence. In practice, this does not hold up. Some governments prescribe for us, in legislation, which children we should prefer if we use IVF. This is, for instance, the case in the U.K. There are also situations, in which medical professionals put pressure on people, for example, to either undergo sterilization or terminate a pregnancy. Some professionals are very good at making people feel that they are stupid if they don't (want to) go along with the given advice.

The technological advances that have made it all possible are now moving much faster than most of us realize. In theory, we will soon be able to order our children according to our detailed specifications, pick their properties from a catalog. To some degree, this is already the case but not all of it will be possible because genes often are not binary either/or switches.

The new eugenics goes by various other names, such as personal eugenics, private eugenics, liberal eugenics, and consumer eugenics. Other terms that are associated with the new eugenics are PGD, PGS, genetic screening, egg (donor) selection, procreative beneficence, sperm (donor) selection, pre-embryo (de)selection, embryo (de)selection, positive or negative selection, IVF, (ex-ante) human enhancement, (ex-ante) bioenhancement, (ex-ante) cognitive enhancement, (ex-ante) moral enhancement and a few more.

There is also, of course, the phrase "designer babies", which most people do not define when they use it. Some people use it in an exaggerated way with the apparent intention to ridicule anyone who has the guts to dare ask questions or voice doubts. I define designer baby as any baby that is chosen over another baby that is or would be viable and would live into adulthood.

IVF once started out as a way of helping couples who couldn't get pregnant, but now is increasingly used to postpone pregnancy to allow women to have careers. While IVF still has a low success rate, it is a flourishing commercial practice nevertheless. In their 2015 publication "Infertility around the globe: new thinking on gender, reproductive technologies and global movements in the 21st century", Inhorn and Patrizio reported that while only 45 of the 191 World Health Organization's member states had IVF services in the year 2000, the number had risen to 59 five years later and to 105 another five years later. More than half of these clinics were located in Japan and India. Nine Middle Eastern countries were among the 48 countries carrying out the highest number of IVF cycles per million inhabitants.

So if you thought, as I once did, that the use of such assisted reproductive technologies (ART) is greatest in the United States, you were wrong. Europe was leading the list at 56% of conducted aspirations (egg harvesting), but this was not exclusively concentrated in its richest countries. (The order from lowest to highest was Moldova - Poland - Hungary – Montenegro - Macedonia - Portugal - Lithuania - Albania – Austria - Ireland - Ukraine – Germany - United Kingdom – Croatia – Italy - Cyprus - France - Switzerland - the Netherlands - Serbia - Spain - Estonia - Czech Republic - Finland - Norway - Slovenia - Sweden - Iceland - Denmark - Belgium.) It was followed by Asia at 23%, with North America including Canada in third place at 15%. (See the 2015 publication by Präg and Mills.) The only geographical areas that had no or very limited IVF or other ART services available were sub-Saharan Africa and most of Central Asia. These were also areas with high secondary infertility – after the first child – partly due to botched (illegal) abortions.

There is some speculation that the use of ART is sometimes promoted to boost low fertility numbers to ensure that a country's population continues to grow, even though IVF does not actually have much effect on a country's fertility at the moment. In view of the burden that population growth places on our habitat, you could question how responsible such a practice would be.

In Britain, about 100 women per day ask for IVF (36,500 women) and roughly 50,000 women per year undergo IVF treatment (2017). Britons also go abroad for IVF. Depending on where in the U.K. you live, IVF is publicly financed in the U.K. for those who are eligible. In 2017, only 35% of the IVF treatments in England were paid for by the National

Health Service whereas 62% were paid for in Scotland, according to the U.K.'s Human Fertilisation and Embryology Authority (HFEA).

People in the U.S. and other countries may be quick to assume that funded healthcare provision is the same throughout the U.K. and that just about anything is paid for. In reality, your postcode within one of the countries in the United Kingdom can even determine what medication you will get, the newest or an older, less effective one.

Many couples in the U.K. spend £15,000 to £50,000 on IVF. IVF is also expensive in the United States (around $10,000 per cycle, excluding the medications, which will set you back $2,000 to $4,000) and only possible through private insurance. In some other countries, IVF and similar forms of ART are much less expensive. A Belgian-led non-profit organization recently invented an IVF method that costs only €200 per cycle.

IVF is currently actually still relatively unsuccessful, but this is bound to change with technological progress and the experience that is being gained worldwide. Particularly in China, the use of PGD to de-select certain embryos has been sky-rocketing. Eventually, the effects on society of selecting the properties of offspring will kick in, and to some degree, they already have. (Deselection of female fetuses and of fetuses with Down syndrome is changing some countries' populations.)

In addition, we now have techniques for editing genomes. This can be done in a way that affects only one individual (somatic), but can also be applied in a way that theoretically results in changes in all offspring (germline). (Watch Renée Wegrzyn's talk if you want to learn more about possible safeguards and ways to correct mistakes; see Videos).

So far, CRISPR is mainly being looked at in a way that does not "edit out" people but protects them against developing serious physical conditions as adults. In the west, we have not allowed this to lead to actual babies yet because there are still too many questions to be answered to expose non-consenting humans to the risks.

In 2019, however, many bioethics experts as well as many scientists and legal scholars were shocked to hear the news from China that two human babies (Lulu and Nana) had been experimented on with CRISPR and had been allowed to be born, illegally. The babies' genomes had been tweaked in such a way that the babies are now supposedly immune

## Eugenics, old and new

to HIV. This also affects other properties, however, and it's not clear yet how this is going to pan out in practice.

It called global attention to the fact that there is an urgent need for a global guideline for these new techniques. Among other things, the news from China resulted in leading scientists calling for a global moratorium. So did leading bioethicists, founders of companies like CRISPR Therapeutics and many other people. In November 2019, the director of the National Institutes of Health (NIH) in the U.S. also spoke out in favor of such a global moratorium. By then, the U.S. House of Representatives had reinstated such a ban for the U.S., after briefly having lifted it, which in itself indicates how complicated the decision-making in this area is and how conflicted the decision-makers are. The scientist in question, He Jankui, was sentenced to three years in prison. In the meantime, a third CRISPR baby appears to have been born in China, also created by He.

So we really do need to talk about this, sooner rather than later.

**We need to talk about this**

## 4. Why we need to talk about this

"All the elements for your happiness are already here. There's no need to run, strive, search or struggle. Just be."

– Thích Nhất Hạnh

This is not about whether you are against or for progress in science and technology.

We might end up wrecking the good life if we were to proceed full steam ahead with the little we know right now. If we allow the unbridled application of germline modification of embryos by using techniques like CRISPR, right now, with the little we know now, we might end up demolishing society.

We might not.

If we do, then that mistake will be likely impossible to correct.

We may think that we have enough safeguards in place, but we won't know whether we really do until after we've come to depend on those safeguards.

When you look back into history, you will notice that we've often been completely unable to predict any negative effects of what we saw as awesome scientific and technological progress. Sometimes, we overlooked things that are blatantly obvious in hindsight and I am still scratching my head over how the heck we managed to do that. We've even given a Nobel Prize in medicine for one of an invention that backfired badly, namely DDT. In other cases, such as that of thalidomide, its disastrous effects were ignored for the sake of profits. (See Chapter 11 for more about this.) A lot of it we were simply completely unable to predict. A recent bit of scientific news was that ibuprofen affects male fertility in humans. Would you have foreseen that?

So let's look into this some more.

First, concerning the use of genome-editing techniques such as CRISPR, we need to make a distinction between interventions that only affect the individual in question and interventions that (theoretically) will also be present in offspring and may not be reversible.

The first concerns so-called somatic cells. Alterations are made to DNA in cells that are not part of human reproduction hence do not get passed on, but can cure a disease such as when these cells do not make a protein that the body needs to be able to function well.

Interventions that will be passed on to offspring are called germline modifications.

The use of CRISPR appears to be a form of human enhancement.

I see no major problem with people who want to CRISPR themselves just like I don't want people to criticize the fact that I would love to be able to run on grass again every day, like I used to, or that one of the first things I do in the morning is to make a nice mug of strong coffee. This is along the lines of whether or not you take a painkiller, which kind and how many or whether you should eat anything containing peanuts if you have a nut allergy.

Human enhancement is something we all do. When you have a mug of Java before you go for a run or when you're working late, you do this because the coffee enhances your capabilities at that point. It makes you a "better" person for a while, better within the scope of what you want to achieve at that point. Caffeine is also a bronchodilator, so if you have mild asthma, your coffee will give you a double boost.

The element of risk plays a role, along with questions about a person's free will and freedom to make decisions for oneself. We all take risks on a daily basis, even when we open the front door. We take risks when we drive our cars and take public transport.

Is the practice of pre-embryo, sperm and egg selection based on (genetic) characteristics as a form of human enhancement? I feel that it is not. There is no attempt to change anything if an embryo or fetus is not chosen or aborted. It is pure discrimination, preferring one person over another, as harsh as it may sound. I suppose that that would be old-style eugenics, then.

The use of CRISPR in ART concerns the enhancement of a non-consenting human, however. There is a big difference between doing

## Why we need to talk about this 27

something to yourself and doing something to another being. This is a crucial difference; I will come back to this in Chapters 7 and 8.

Using CRISPR to cure (prevent) serious health conditions is one thing. But what happens when parents tweak properties of children that do not result in the remediation of a health condition? Take an imaginary case in which parents tweak what would have become a brown-eyed, brown-haired girl and end up with a red-headed girl with green eyes. Would that be a different person than the girl with the brown eyes and brown hair would have been? Or could we say that the brown-haired brown-eyed girl became enhanced, even though this would be a matter of personal taste?

I don't know how to answer that question. I have experimented a little bit with my own external properties and it is both fun and amazing to see how differently people respond to you on the basis of hair color alone or on how you dress, but also quite shocking. How we are treated does influence us. Does that turn us into different people? Perhaps not, but it can determine a lot of our behavior and our opportunities, so it certainly influences how we live our lives.

How would you feel if a stranger walked up to you on the street and started cutting your hair out of the blue?

The problem with this is that you haven't given consent. (Let's not go into the legal intricacies of consent and the need for reform.) That is a major problem of using CRISPR in ART. Something is being done to you that you probably cannot change and will likely be stuck with for the rest of your life and for which you cannot give consent.

What kind of risk do those children run? (That is, apart from the scientific/technological risks inherent in the use of these new technologies, such as that one gene can code for several properties so that removing one can also introduce health risks.)

Well, for one, these people could end up having been modified according to fashion trends that put them at a disadvantage as adults. As Hank Greely, a law professor who specializes in bioethics at Stanford, has pointed out, the people who got the first nose jobs ended up regretting them badly when the type of nose they had chosen went out of fashion. Breast augmentations have gone through a similar fashion cycle.

In an interview with Dutch TV, bioethicist Julian Savulescu offered the theoretical example that parents might want to control whether or not their child is going to be gay if they are living in a society in which gays are persecuted. That situation, however, could be wildly different by the time that youngster reaches puberty. These parents would have chosen a way to eradicate their own worries. They would not have asked the child what the child wanted.

In the discussion about designer babies, also the topic of height sometimes crops up as an example to discuss. There have been studies that seem to indicate that the taller you are, the more successful you are in life. There are countries in which people are undergoing complicated procedures so that they can become taller, just like there are Asian people who undergo surgery to make their eyes appear more western.

When you look into it in more depth, you may find that this successfulness is probably not determined by height, but by childhood nutrition and the associated benefits of that as well as by the nature of the society in which people are living, which values those societies hold high (according to, for example, Hofstede's system, or whether these values are western and capitalist/materialistic or not).

Dutch young people are now increasingly often signing up for surgeries that limit their height because they are, for example, fed up with bumping their heads in doorways. The Dutch are the tallest people on earth and this appears to be a result of plenty of dairy in the children's diets in combination with the fact that they are growing up in a prosperous, egalitarian society, in which there is no massive deep poverty like in the U.K.

So shouldn't we rather be creating more egalitarian societies and eradicate childhood poverty instead of contemplating the tweaking of genes that make children grow into taller adults?

Moreover, taller people put a higher environmental burden on the planet, have higher costs of living and are at risk for certain health conditions. They may also have shorter life spans.

So you could just as easily argue for tweaking genomes to encourage a form of dwarfism that does not compromise health. You could use social media marketing to make dwarfism attractive. I am not saying that we should, simply attempting to show that most advocates of any way of being (being taller, being smarter) have a bias that makes them ignore certain facts, simply because they are not looking for those facts, and that you could just as easily argue for the opposite.

A similar discussion can be had about whether or not to increase the IQ of one's offspring. It is not true that the higher your IQ is, the happier you are. A high IQ does not make you immune to assaults or robberies or diseases like progressive MS or traffic accidents or even against breaking a leg when out skiing or horse-riding. IQ is a western, capitalistic value that a lot of people associate with high income and they take high income or rather, socioeconomic status, as a person's true measure.

Where would it stop? Would it stop with people who are 4 meters tall so that they could be considered more successful than the people who are 3 meters tall? Would it stop at an IQ of 300, which you can only accomplish if you keep average IQ right where it is, as IQ is a relative measure? The latter would, therefore, go hand in hand with increased inequality.

Would only the grandchildren of Bill Gates, Jeff Bezos, Arron Banks and Donald Trump be allowed to tweak their offspring, in practice? Or should we make it free and unlimited for all future parents?

What risks might society run if we were to allow germline application of techniques like CRISPR on embryos and newborns freely, given the little we know right now?

Again, this is aside from the inherent medical risks and so on, such as the fact that if you code for one desired property you often also code for an undesired property or get rid of another desired property (and aside from the fact that the tweaking the way I describe it here may never be possible in exactly this way).

I think that the greater risk is to society at large. If we proceed too rapidly we could be dissolving the glue that keeps societies together.

Medical insurance – as Michael Sandel has pointed out previously; if I recall correctly – was initially based on solidarity. Though this is often no longer the case, sadly, the idea behind insurance is that we all pay in and bear the burden of some people's medical misfortune together. Sandel is not happy with the idea of humans wanting to create perfect humans. In his article "The case against perfection" published in the Atlantic in 2004, Michael Sandel (who was a member of the U.S.

President's Council on Bioethics at the time) referred to (social) solidarity within this context. If fate no longer controls most of our destiny, it becomes harder and harder to feel solidarity toward others, he argued.

I share that concern, but I make a distinction between inclusive solidarity, which I often refer to as "the glue that binds society" and exclusive solidarity (protectionism).

If there is enough to go around, for everyone, if nobody needs to fear a shortage, if there is abundance in a society and everyone feels provided for, it is much easier for people to feel generous toward strangers, people who aren't part of the in-group. That's what I call inclusive solidarity. When times are tough, people tend to restrict feelings of solidarity to their own group and exclude strangers. I call that exclusive solidarity. So-called old boys' networks are examples of exclusive solidarity.

The new eugenics may (initially) encourage exclusive solidarity, the selective protection of "our kind of people" over the protection of others. It could lead to the deliberate creation of different classes of human beings, a theme that was explored in the film Gattaca and also features in the novel "The ultimate brainchild" by Richard Bintanja. It is possible that this would eventually be evened out again, but we have no way of looking into the future to see how the unrestricted application of consumer eugenics would work out for our grandchildren's children and their children.

Frances Kamm (who just like Sandel is based at Harvard University) has argued that a parent's unconditional love includes seeking better attributes for a child, in her 2005 comment on Sandel's 2004 article in the Atlantic. That reminds me of what Joseph Connolly describes in his work "Style" and I consider attribute-seeking in contradiction with unconditional love. The attributes are not sought for the child but for the parent(s).

Unconditional love means that you'll love the child (person) as he or she is, with no condition attached. Kamm's unconditional love, by contrast, seems to refer to the efforts and sacrifices a parent may be willing to make for the sake of their child. That is not the same. Unconditional love on the condition that a child complies with how the parents want the child to be, that is unconditional possessiveness.

Kamm, too, saw that the idea of seeking "better" attributes is

### Why we need to talk about this 31

problematic and came up with a concept she called sufficientarianism, which does not seek perfection but merely what is sufficient. This appears to suffer from the same problem. Who determines what is sufficient? Kamm, however, realized that as well. Next, she asked "...could we really safely alter people, not making disastrous mistakes?" and commented: "A deeper issue, I think, is our lack of imagination as designers." Her concern was that "people will focus on too simple and basic a set of" what they consider good qualities. This is linked to the idea that parents might end up choosing what happens to be trendy at the time of choosing.

That is easy enough to solve, in theory. If, for example, there is a gene for musical talent, you could decide to give everyone that gene. If there are genes for being good at chess or good at basketball, you could give those to everyone as well.

At this point, I feel that I have to point out once again, keeping certain scientists in mind, that I am not talking about whether or not this will be possible. That is not what this book is about. I want more people to think about and discuss the principle of doing such things, what the advantages and disadvantages could be and whether other approaches could be more effective, but I have seen what, for example, some professors in genetics have to say when non-geneticists start talking about what geneticists seem to feel is exclusively their field. This is a discussion about our lives and about the world we live in.

In her comment, Kamm also wrote that in her eyes, the duty to help others has to do with respect and concern for the values of other persons, regardless of whether or not we believe that they are to blame for the situation they are in. This was a comment on Sandel's view that the more chance – fate – there is in our life choices, the more reason we have to share our fate with others (inclusive solidarity).

Until I heard neuroscientist Rebecca Saxe speak about the neuroscience of hate (see "Videos" in "Sources of information" at the end of the book), I believed that inclusive solidarity is largely based on whether we can identify with other people or not.

Indeed, fate has something to do with that, as Michael Sandel has said. If we can see that we are all slaves to fate, it is easier to recognize that we're all in the same boat.

But it's more complicated than that. There is something that underlies whether or not we are able to identify with someone.

It is related to how secure people feel. They automatically translate other people's bad luck to what it means for themselves and how secure they feel determines how they see this. They subconsciously ask themselves whether the same bad luck could strike them too and if so, how they would like the people around them to respond.

Rebecca Saxe made me realize where some of this insecurity of insecurity comes from (but not all). When people feel that there is not enough of the good stuff to go around, they become less likely to share it with strangers, with people that they do not identify with. That's sheer biology. So if they can identify with the other person, they will want to help that unfortunate soul, but if they don't identify at all, then they won't. The greater the degree of inequality, the smaller the chance is that a person is able to identify with someone else.

What Saxe had to say fits with what social epidemiologist Richard Wilkinson (see "Videos" in "Sources of information" at the end of the book) has been saying as well, namely that everyone in society benefits from greater equality, even those at the top.

As a consequence, we should be striving to create maximum equality in society, by which I mean that – among other things – we should eradicate the kind of deep poverty that determines what kind of adults children can grow into.

I do not see this as an alternative for the use of CRISPR in ART but as a condition for its continued use. These two developments should go hand in hand and feed back into each other.

I don't see equality in terms of "declaring everyone synonymous" but in terms of allowing everyone to flourish to the best of their abilities and personal wishes (provided the latter does not harm anyone).

To bring it closer to home, let's look at the example of male-on-female rape. Any woman of any age can get raped in any kind of situation or environment, but when a woman gets raped, a mechanism kicks in among many men and also among many other women that assesses other women's chances of getting raped and their own measure of powerlessness. It is reassuring to be able to tell yourself that you would never get raped or that your sister would never get raped and one way in

## Why we need to talk about this 33

which you can do that is by blaming the victim. Because you or your sister would never do that, hence you are safe and your sister is safe because "rape only happens to women who do something wrong".

"She should have been dressed differently." "She should have been home at that hour." "She should not have gone to that neighborhood." "She should not have worn lipstick." "She should not have had this many boyfriends." "She should have had a boyfriend." "She shouldn't have gone alone." "She should not have had dancing as a hobby." In spite of the "me too" wave, the blame mechanism is still alive and kicking with regard to male-on-female rape.

This same mechanism exists in many other instances of "bad luck".

Within the context of the new eugenics, however, we have to be very careful not to equate "bad luck" with "having a child that does not fulfill our wishes". Having a girl in your own country or flying to another country so that you can have the desired male baby is not about "bad luck". It is about seeing your baby as a product, the way you would purchase a matching chair that fits neatly in the corner of the room and completes the set or buy a painting to add to the collection of artworks.

I think that these non-technological challenges of the new eugenics are considerable. I think that we should also take it slow for that reason and give everyone a chance to weigh in on this discussion. We have made so many mistakes in the past when we enthusiastically jumped on the bandwagon of progress, only to find later that we'd been shooting ourselves in the foot. With our increasing scientific and technological powers also comes a greater chance that we do something very competently yet with such a scale of consequences that we end up regretting it badly, even more so then we've already done. (We've wrecked our own habitat, people, and while we are curing diseases after disease, we are also making ourselves sicker and sicker. We are clearly still missing something, still doing too many things that are not the right things.)

I find it worrisome that the new eugenics runs the risk of turning children into products that have to meet certain expectations of parents. Of course, that parents have expectations for their children and that this can lead to excesses is nothing new. It was what inspired London-based author Joseph Connolly to write a bulky novel called "Style"; it was described as a "brilliant exposition of maniacal parental ambition within a society in thrall to celebrity and fashionable acquisition" and published in 2015.

Real life promptly followed this up with the college admission scandal in the U.S. Rich parents had been paying "designer label" schools under the table to get the schools to admit their children. It does not give me the impression that these parents had a lot of faith in their children, and I don't see bribing schools for your children as an expression of unconditional love either. Speaking of seeking better attributes for one's children...

I think that the unrestrained creation of children according to specifications could increasingly skew parental expectations and ambitions and might push them out of control, not just for a few individual parents, but as a general trend. This could hollow out the most-valued principle of parenthood, the concept of unconditional love, and this is closely tied to inclusive solidarity. Allowing the deterioration of the unconditional love parents (should) have for children and risking its eventual disappearance could have seriously deleterious consequences for humanity as it is the glue that keeps us all together. How would we make decisions in a cohesion-less world? Could we start seeing each other as enemies? Could we collectively move toward increasingly psychopathic societies – a trend that has already been detected – and if so, what might this look like in practice? Is it something we must avoid or would we see the development of a new kind of order that might actually work very well?

We don't know. There is no way for us to know.

Traditional parenthood itself can be replaced. Commune life, kibbutzim and other alternative forms of living have shown that. You could turn parenting into a profession; you could attach licensing to parenthood.

In fact, there is another fascinating technological development that may end up solving many issues and steer our lives in a completely different direction. We will no longer have traditional gestation at some point. Women will no longer have to get pregnant, which would likely in itself also remove some of the unconditional love that most parents feel for their children.

Maybe we will lovingly grow our babies in cute little incubation pods at home. Perhaps having children will become a privilege or a duty with

## Why we need to talk about this

which only certain individuals will be tasked, the way we now task people with great IT skills with using those skills instead of telling them to go out to sea in boats and catch fish for our supermarkets.

Maybe babies will be created centrally and handed out to approved parents. In an interview for Dutch TV, bioethicist Julian Savulescu suggested that assigning children (embryos) to people randomly might be a good solution. The combination of these two ideas could be all we need to preserve unconditional love.

That may also be the time when we can safely and freely apply genetic selection and genome editing and gene therapy and, yes, have a more product-like view of children. I would still like this to be one that puts a duty to nourish and care on the shoulders of the parents and carers, instead of putting a duty to perform on the shoulders of the children.

This development of artificial uteruses (artificial wombs, which already have been used successfully for sheep) will also settle all discussions on the topic of abortion, thankfully. In September 2023, the news that the FDA was considering clinical trials for artificial wombs hit the media. It held a meeting on the question whether the technology might be ready to save younger "preemies". Artificial wombs for humans are not yet suitable for gestation from conception.

By the time we grow children in pods, a lot more will have changed in society. I hope that by then, all kinds of men and women will get to eat their lab-grown honey mustard chicken filets, if they want honey mustard chicken for dinner, no matter what good or bad luck they may have had. I hope that by then, all real-life chickens will get to live their lives as free as a bird again, too.

**We need to talk about this**

# 5. Bias

*"Congress acknowledged that society's accumulated myths and fears about disability and disease are as handicapping as are the physical limitations that flow from actual impairment."*
– Justice William J. Brennan, Jr., School Bd. of Nassau, Fl. v. Arline, 480 U.S. 273 (1973)

In this chapter, I use the word "bias" in the sense of "rigidly sticking to one's own skewed opinion, usually without being aware of it", and particularly concerning stuff that we all experience, the kind of stuff that essentially represents the huge range of diversity in the human population. In case you didn't know that yet: We all have stuff.

Social media are helping us uncover how broad this range is, this range of stuff we call diversity. Would you have predicted that it is possible to disagree on whether a dress is black with blue or white with gold, for example? Did you know that for someone with a severe nut allergy, even one bite into a meal can lead to severe brain damage? That too, is diversity, as are gifts like synesthesia, altruism, compassion and even the lack of emotional – but not cognitive – empathy.

Years after I started writing the first edition of this book, I learned that it is metabolically disadvantageous for the human brain to try to have empathy for what it is not familiar with. This is extremely helpful because most of us also tend to be biased toward others who seem to lack empathy. I also learned that this is often simply because they have empathy for different groups of people, which we then fail to see. From this, I also deduce that it is good to be surrounded by as much diversity as possible. This is confirmed by the finding that companies with the greatest diversity do best. People simply get along better and people who get along better perform better. Diverse environments are more fun.

Diversity is all around us, every day, and there is a heck of a lot more of this than we used to be aware. That's because we used to focus on mostly very obvious differences in outward appearances. It seems to be an expression of the phenomenon known as the focusing illusion.

Diversity is a huge multidimensional space in which we all take up a unique spot. It may even be helpful to think of it as a universe, with time warps and spots where space folds back onto itself.

If you want to experience how bias based on external attributes works, carry out a few simple experiments. It's usually not only a great learning opportunity but also a fun experience. Change your appearance, big time. If you're normally dressed in a relatively business-like or middle-of-the-road manner, get yourself an eye-catching coat, for example, one that is a shiny silver or a vibrant pink or turquoise if you're a man. A huge one, with a lot of fabric, so that you really stand out. If you're a woman and don't usually do this, color your hair blue, purple, green or pink or get yourself a wig in one of those colors. You could also dress as if you are homeless. Get frumpy clothes from a thrift store or charity shop (and wear white trainers if you're in the U.K.). You could get dorky glasses. Wear a beanie or a hat. Just wearing a hat or a cap can already change how people respond to you. Travel on trains, trams and busses. Go to cash machines, into banks, into theaters, museums, restaurants, all the usual places that you go to. Go have an espresso or cappuccino at Costa if you're in the U.K. or walk into your local sit-down Krispy Kreme or Papa John's, go shopping at the Bijenkorf in Amsterdam or walk into a jewelry store.

Diversity is seen as negative when it equals adversity – such as colon cancer or breast cancer affecting several relatives – or when it causes adversity as a result of stigmatization and discrimination as a result of extreme bias.

I can see two main reasons for the existence of bias:

- Living or growing up in a bubble, resulting in unfamiliarity with what else is "out there";
- Insecurity, such as resulting from socioeconomic inequality.

Socioeconomic inequality creates a sense that there is not enough of a resource to go around. This makes people defensive, wanting to protect their own. It's biology. I learned that from Rebecca Saxe's talk (see "Videos" in "Sources of information" at the end of the book).

Insecurity can also come from upset with what has happened to someone else and not wanting it to happen to ourselves or loved ones, as I've explained in the previous chapter. That's why people can feel the need to look for blame, explanations that result in the reassurance that the same thing could never happen to us or to our loved ones because we would not do anything that might result in it or we would be smart enough or strong enough to avoid it or get away unscathed.

Equality – viewing everyone's lives as equally important – has a lot to do with respect. This is not the respect in the sense of being impressed by someone's accomplishments in an area or someone's socioeconomic status, but an acknowledgment that all beings share very similar needs and deserve to be free from certain things, such as violence and bullying. We all have certain requirements, such as for food, sleep and shelter, and we all deserve to live in peace and live our lives in a manner of our own choosing, provided the way we live does not harm others.

Bias can result in not treating other people with an equal measure of human respect. Bias also has to do with stereotyping, and ultimately stigmas and discrimination. Stereotypes usually contain an element of truth but do not allow much room for the variability within a group of people. An example could be something along the lines of "women are better at cleaning kitchens" and "men are bad at cleaning kitchens". A related stigma could be that women are considered of no use other than for cleaning kitchens. Discrimination would then result in women not being hired for any jobs that do not involve the cleaning of kitchens. This is one example of how non-mainstream people can be held back by society and become "disabled" by society.

Another type of disablement by society occurs because we focus our society on people who are average and forget to take others into account. We tend to focus on people who are like us and often more or less forget that others exist as well. We tend to value what we know because we are don't know what we are not familiar with. It would be impossible for me to say whether it would be wonderful for people who use a wheelchair to live on the moon as I have never used a wheelchair and have no idea whether less gravity would make it easier or harder to use a wheelchair. Personally, I don't like electronic displays in green letters and numbers, specifically if they are at some distance because I find them hard to read.

For centuries, we built buildings with steps and staircases, excluding and handicapping everyone who's unable to negotiate them independently. We still stuff neurologically atypical people in institutions where they are kept like prisoners and still too often abused. We deprive them of all opportunities because we still have a lot of learning and catching up to do on how to treat all beings with the respect they deserve and what this would look like in practice.

Equality is not about pretending that everyone is a beautiful male peacock. Equality is about acknowledging the beauty in everyone and for example noticing how gorgeous starlings are and how varied their song and what skilled fliers they are, even though they don't display a huge fan of impossibly gorgeous feathers, the way male peacocks do and admitting that there is nothing wrong with being a female peacock either.

Equality is about losing our obsession with male peacocks and with superlatives. Equality is about accepting that the art of being is enough, acknowledging that being alive is enough. Equality is about accepting that there is no such thing as a measure of worthiness, hence that everyone is equally deserving. It is not about forcing everyone to be the same. It is about enabling everyone to be the best they can be, as defined by themselves.

The wish to tweak our offspring and create designer babies of any kind is related to the lack of this type of respect in society. If every human being had the same opportunities, the same chance of ending up fulfilled and contented, if everyone would be allowed to be who they are, there might be no more wish at all for parents to want to give their offspring certain characteristics because it would make no difference. It would also mean that parents would be able to get all the support they might need.

It is sad to hear someone say something along the lines of "Yes, I have progressive MS and my life's become pretty shitty but at least I have enough money to carry out any adaptations that I need." Think of what it means for all the people with progressive MS who do not have the kind of money that makes it possible to adapt their living surroundings or move house and have the house adapted before moving in. This plays a big factor in the considerations of the new eugenics too.

If you read that a child with cerebral palsy who rides horses, plays music and does many other things has not been able to go to school for 20 months because none of the schools are suitable for the child's wheelchair or an autistic child cannot go to school because the trip on the buses would take 90 minutes one way and no other transport is available because the child has turned 16, it is crystal-clear that society is still far from inclusive and that it is still society that creates many hindrances.

Even the factors of which we think that they make people more successful often turn out to be related to socioeconomic inequality. We seem to have forgotten that we began businesses and professions not in order to accumulate as much money as possible but to be of service to each other, and use one's talents best to that end. Money and fame – earning power – became the measuring sticks along which we assess a human being's true value.

At the same time, we started mass-producing products. We began rejecting products with flaws, not just at the end of the production lines but also in the fruit and vegetable aisles at the supermarkets. It caused us to assess humans that way too, as if they have to meet manufacturing specs and as if there is such a thing as a standard for human beings that we need to meet.

This view also still dominates among medical professionals. It is reflected in what insurance companies will pay for (surgery to make someone resemble that standard more versus anything that works just as well or better but that leaves people whole as who they are, that accepts that they do not fit the mold) and in the legislation that forbids people to implant an embryo that does not meet the specs.

It is highly significant that only a minority of deaf parents are interested in deliberately producing a deaf child and that this is usually called a "diminishment". We should see it as enhancement because that is what it is in the eyes of those parents. There is no such thing as a "diminished" human being and to suggest that there is should give us pause. A person is either human or not. There is no such thing as being a diminished human.

So what shall we do with the new eugenics? Should we ban it altogether?

I don't think so.

But I do believe that we need to take a step back and take it slow and that we have to let it happen in conjunction with these other badly needed changes (greater inclusivity among humans, less focus on consumerism, better care for our environment, greater compassion for non-human animals). I also believe that we need to reach a global consensus so that we can legislate for the new eugenics globally, as national legislation is fairly useless if anyone can simply travel to another country to circumvent one's own country's laws.

And I want you to think about the following. Why not add genes that will allow you to walk on four legs and be as fast as a jaguar? Why not add genes that will make you grow wings? Would you want those of pigeon or those of a pelican? Would you like to be dependent on another human to remove the protective sheaths in which new feathers develop? That's what birds are doing when they preen each other. What are your arguments for and against doing any of these things? Why not surgically implant wheels under our feet to make us faster? Why not make everyone autistic? Why not implant fish genes that make our skin a fluorescent green or pink? It's been done to cats and other mammals. Wouldn't it be wonderful to pick your skin color in the morning? Would you like to go purple tomorrow, with golden specks and dashes of pink? Just for fun?

If you look at ongoing trends of emancipation (Chapter 11, Appendix C), you will see that some variations of humans have started to do astoundingly well, after we stopped depriving those people of normal human contact and of normal human life experiences. When we, as society, stop disabling people but start enabling them, great things are possible. We've seen that happen with women, too. As we are nowhere near the end of that learning curve yet, it might be a bit too soon to start tweaking our offspring and correct "defects" that aren't defects.

Some of the problems we may think we are solving with the new eugenics do not stem from the supposed limitations that human diversity represents. The problem is our collective failure to accept that humans who are not 100% like ourselves are equally worthy of life and are equally valuable. The problem is our inability to see beyond our own limitations. (That's bias, yes.)

But there is even more.

Many of the arguments given for doing away with a lot of variety among humans may dissolve in the future, for example, because science and technologies will come up with creative ways to make all people's lives easier. We already have people who use their brains to operate machinery (artificial arms) and we are developing exoskeletons that can make a huge difference for some people.

## Bias

In future societies, we will also all have a lot more time on our hands as increasingly more of the "money-making" will be done by intelligent machines. That would take away a large chunk of the motivation behind the new eugenics in the consumerist, career-enhancing sense. It would also mean that we will have much more time to look after one another properly.

**We need** to talk about this

# 6. Brain-based conditions

*"Few people are capable of expressing with equanimity opinions which differ from the prejudices of their social environment. Most people are incapable of forming such opinions."*

– Albert Einstein

If you look into brain-based variations of human life that express themselves as a wide range of different mental abilities and patterns of behavior, you will find that this space is as multidimensional as physical health but is dealt with very differently. It has not gotten the amount of research that physical health has received and it is riddled with stigmas and embarrassment. Many of these different states of being are fine. Some of them can cause problems, as with physical health issues that do not affect behavior.

Before I continue, let me make clear that by "mental abilities", I do not mean "IQ".

It is odd that we still divide health into physical health and "mental" health, even though the two are inseparable and that mental health is mostly related to one organ, namely the brain. However, the use of the word "mental" suggests that people are to blame for the makeup of their brains. It is related to the word "mentality", after all.

Along with many others, I sometimes wonder why we insist on the continued development of psychiatric taxonomies that seem to serve no other purpose than that it enables us to label people and place them in a box. It is such a subjective art, this kind of diagnosis, that many people continue to be diagnosed with conditions that they don't have and are fed medications that do more harm than good. Sometimes it feels like just about everything that is part of the human condition is being called a "disorder" nowadays.

Some specialists say that children are now sometimes being "diagnosed" with attention deficit hyperactivity disorder (ADHD) because they are – are you ready for this? – merely still young. That indicates that something is really going in the wrong direction in this field. Young children behave differently because they are young children. I can't help but wonder if the increasing incidence of ADHD may (also) reflect an increasing emphasis on the medical "standardization" of humans and/or the fact that our educational system has not undergone much innovation for a long time and is inherently stifling for many children.

The creative genius behind the musical "Cats" might have been given the diagnosis of ADHD if she had been young now, Ken Robinson has said (see "Videos" in "Sources of information" at the end of the book). She was believed to be learning-disabled and was sent for an assessment. Thankfully, she was examined by the right professional who correctly identified her as simply not being what I call a desk jockey. If she hadn't been that lucky, she might never have been allowed to develop her talents. As the sedentary lifestyle many of us are forced to lead these days is severely detrimental to our health – the human body was not designed to spend the majority of time on or in a chair – many people who are (mis)diagnosed with ADHD may well be physically fitter and healthier than the rest of us. We also have a global epidemic of depression, which is the cause of a great deal of disability. So we're clearly doing something wrong at the moment, but we worry much more about swine flu and bird flu.

I feel tempted to advise mental health professionals to watch as many videos of elephants as they can and to watch at least one per day if they can. Videos of young ones, older ones, free ones, and ones that are miserable – mentally ill – in captivity and who may even have been physically abused and those who are then taken to for example the Global Elephant Sanctuary in Brazil where they tend to bounce back remarkably as well as videos of elephants who are mourning the loss of a family member or friend and perhaps a few videos shared by The Dodo as well.

Maybe we should do away with the mental health professions and start all over. A study published in 2019 found that most research published by psychologists and psychiatrists is biased. That's worrisome. This means that many people are being "treated" on the basis of the research equivalent of fake news.

We, as society, still often abuse people who aren't neurotypical. Whether they are gay or autistic, bipolar or schizophrenic, were abused as

## Brain-based conditions 47

children and have PTSD or DID, or have dissenting political opinions because they are smart, we still often lock them up, tie them up, beat them up and put them in chains. We also taser them and wrestle them to the floor, sometimes killing them in the process, not just in places like Indonesia and some countries in Africa but also in places like the Netherlands, New Zealand and the U.K. Research has also found that people whose skins are lily-white are much less likely to get tasered. Tasering is predominantly used on people who aren't white and on people with brain-based conditions.

This may be the result of the fact that we are all biological creatures and often respond with the "crocodile" part of the brain. Our fight-flight-freeze mechanism engages when we encounter manifestations of other people's brain-based conditions or people who look slightly different than the people we grew up with. We may see behaviors that are out of the ordinary for us. They may cross important boundaries, cultural or otherwise. They may make us feel threatened instantly or we may simply not know what to make of it, and that too can make us feel uncomfortable, or threatened, on a very basic level (subliminal). Only in rare cases do we have good reason to feel threatened, however. Watch the Pixar/Disney short movie "Loop" as particularly the YouTube video about the making of "Loop" to help you bring this in focus (see "Videos" in "Sources of information" at the end of the book).

Besides the fact that other people's brain-based differences may cause us to try and figure out whether they constitute a danger to us or not, another reason why unfamiliar behaviors make us feel uncomfortable is that they remind us of our own vulnerability. We are all only one stroke, one brain tumor surgery or one bad fall away from a profound personality change. When you see someone behave in a way that you would not want to behave like, this makes you think "this could have been me" even if you are not consciously aware of that thought.

We tend to equate our brains with who we are as if we have total control over what happens in our brains. Most of us have no idea how to do that, however, so why would we expect other people to have full control over what their brains come up with? Some of us meditate and find that this helps greatly. You can use binaural beats to kick your brain into a more relaxed state of being. You can also use binaural beats to kick the brain into a state of fear, though. Kinda makes you think, doesn't it? This may not even work the exact same way for everybody because the different parts of our brains don't all interact in the same way and with the same intensity in different people.

In some people, certain parts of the brain are missing or are much smaller. This can concern the part that has to do with compassion (empathy), the part that gives us what we call "theory of mind". Theory of mind enables us to recognize what may be going on in someone else's mind, for instance, that the person may be in pain or very hungry, or probably very tired and in need of sleep.

The good news is that we used to be convinced that after a certain age, neurons are no longer capable of change or even healing. We also used to be certain that no new neurons are formed after a certain age (early adulthood). This all turned out to be bullshit. It means that we can do a heck of a lot more with, and for, brains than we used to believe. This means that we should at some point in the future be able to do a lot more in terms of healing damaged brains if the people who have such brains would like that. The flexibility of the human brain also means that people can be many different things and that personality is not entirely static.

Want a ridiculously silly example? The way you interact with children and toddlers is very different from how you behave in a tough business negotiation. So are you a pushover or pushy?

Your personality occupies only a small part of the brain. If you compare the brain with a desktop computer, then your personality is formed by the mouse, screen and keyboard (and the beeps from the BIOS). Your personality is your interface with the outside world. A lot more goes on in the processor that is not visible to the outside world and is often not even consciously accessible. (Transcendental meditation, says investor and philanthropist Ray Dalio, can help you access some of the other parts of your brain.)

My own experience is that the other parts of the brain often try to communicate it to me when something is wrong somewhere in my body. The brain receives all that input from all the other parts of the body, of course, and there is also communication going on in the brain, between various parts of the brain. I am not consciously aware of any of this.

I've noticed that when I am unreasonably angry or annoyed and happen to be walking through a building, I will often bump into a doorway or

## Brain-based conditions

cupboard as soon as I think an angry or annoyed thought. It's as if my brain instantly corrects me and says to me "stop it, you're being silly". When I am angry with good reason, this does not happen at all; to the contrary, that kind of anger can make me feel highly focused. It does not mean that every time I bump into something I was angry, but it probably does mean that I was not fully focused on what I was doing in the here and now. Prolonged anger combined with prolonged powerlessness tends to make me depressed. When I am about to come down with a flu, my mood will often tank (though this also has to do with the associated decline in energy). People who have migraines may be able to predict an oncoming migraine attack because of how their mood changes prior to such an attack. Others see light flashes.

When I badly needed a new desk chair and was starting to develop problems in my right wrist, but wasn't aware of the latter yet, I kept bumping notably that elbow into the armrest increasingly hard and increasingly often. My elbow was becoming sore, and so I could no longer ignore it. My brain was trying to tell me that I really needed a new chair, one that was height-adjustable (and one without armrests).

We have a lot of catching up to do in this area that we call mental health. There is still so much knowledge that we don't have, so many questions that we haven't even asked yet. We are only now beginning to discover that structurally different brains with different neural networks can produce structurally different personalities. These structural brain differences show up on brain scans. We're also learning that what goes on in the gut has a big impact on the brain and on behavior. We never expected that, did we?

When such differences result in pathology, maybe we will one day be able to cause the brain to rearrange itself to some degree, get it to grow new neurons and let a few others wither (if the person whose brain it is would like that).

The bad news? We don't know very well yet what to do with brain-based conditions. Not all of them are negative, not at all. Some of them mean that the people who have these conditions suffer by definition, while some other states of being merely require society to be more accommodating and more accepting. Why do we insist that autistic people learn to be like neurotypical people? We don't insist that blind people make themselves see or deaf people make themselves hear. But these different ways of being that we neurotypicals don't quite understand, they tend to scare and confuse us.

People with some states of being such as narcissistic personality disorders, with or without psychopathy, are often vilified, also by mental health professionals and bioethicists. A lot of fear-mongering goes on and a lot of hogwash is flung into the media. In January 2020, I saw a neuroscientist whose name I won't mention tweet about "the dark triad" – which is an old-fashioned term invented by police officers for a condition that does not actually exist as such but works well in films, books and the media – and about "snakes in suits". That kind of sensationalist talk does not contribute to the advancement of the field. If you are in the position that you have to deal with several people with such conditions in your own environment and aren't getting any support, I can forgive you for producing that kind of talk, but it is harder to accept if it is coming from a scientist who is supposed to be searching for explanations and solutions.

Maybe the problem is us, neurotypicals. Maybe the problem is how we see things. What would happen if we decided to see neurodiversity as wealth and as joyful instead of as problematic? What if we started working with that wealth instead of trying to rein it in?

That said, after having resided in southern England for fifteen years, I had no choice but to conclude that most of the English are plain crazy. I am joking, of course, but not quite entirely. Maybe cultural differences are a form of neurodiversity too, something that I just need to learn to accept as well. How do we explain the unusual cases in which people suddenly speak with a strong accent or speak a different language after brain trauma?

Make no mistake, I probably know better than most people that people with personality disorders can be very challenging to deal with and can cause a lot of havoc and confusion. Jokes aside, I learned a few things the hard way after I moved to the U.K. when I had cause to start looking into all sorts of mental health conditions. As a result, I for example discovered that it is easily possible to confuse autism and psychopathy even though they appear to be very different forms of neurodiversity at first sight. Then I discovered that some autism may be related to fear experienced by a pregnant woman after I had already learned that some psychopathy can result from overexposure in the womb to certain

# Brain-based conditions

hormones as a result of living in a war situation and that some children's brains develop psychopathy as a response to repetitive severe abuse. Maybe some "autism" isn't actually autism.

Among other things, I discovered that there was a family in England who was bullied and chased out of their home. (See Charlotte Hayward's article.) Their detailed medical files were sent to their neighbors in the process. Having lived in England for fifteen years, I doubt that the latter happened accidentally. The neighbors did not accept the autism of several members in that family and the local authorities had no idea of how to remedy the situation. That's akin to bullying a family because two members of the family have only one kidney instead of two.

One of my conclusions is that our refusal to accept that these forms of neurodiversity are genuine and that people who have these different brain-based states of being cannot change themselves at will is a huge part of the problem.

Don't ask someone with a narcissistic personality disorder (NPD) to be happy for you with your accomplishments when you know darn well that this is not possible for them. It's foolish. You don't ask a cat to pretend it is a horse either or even ask a Shetland pony to perform like a thin-legged Arabian racehorse and you don't demand that any person will teach himself or herself how to be colorblind either. Instead, you can ask people with NPD for practical advice. Instead, you can learn to separate the silly remarks intended to push your buttons from the gems they also have to offer but tend to hide between their louder words. Not wanting to risk criticism, they may offer you their personal advice or opinion packaged as something that "so and so" said.

It is possible to learn to see that people with these conditions still have their own personalities and learn do disregard the manifestations of the disorders they have. It is possible to see these symptoms like sneezes and coughs. Granted, they can also be much more severe, but that can be the result of a progression that occurred over the years and society's inability to deal with (treat, support) and accept certain conditions.

Some people may realize at a very young age that something about them is different and take courses in psychology to figure out what it is. They may decide that for them to be able to live as peacefully and friction-free as possible, certain environments will be much better than others and they may seek out those environments. In ruthlessly competitive environments, people with NPD are exposed to harsh criticism and they often fare much better among kind people. Others do their best to find professions in which their traits are a plus but through which they can also give something to the world.

Once you start seeing that, a paradigm shift occurs. Most of these people are not "evil" and not "mean-spirited" by nature. There is a Zen saying that talks about "your original face, the face from before your father and mother were born". Maybe that is what it is about.

I think that society may have to focus more on offering opportunities for making the lives of neuro-atypicals easier, thereby making everyone else's lives easier as well. For example, psychopaths seem to need challenges that they consider worthy and rewarding. They are often fearless, which means that they can very quickly become bored. They may need more or different rewards, too. As society, we should be able to come up with opportunities that are tailor-made for them, but such solutions require us to do away with stigmas first. (Please note that I would make an exception for a certain type of psychopath; see video by Real Stories.)

The U.K. government once set out to find psychopaths specifically for major crisis situations in which most of us would likely be sidetracked by our emotions. It became an embarrassment, but such tailor-made approaches do not need to be embarrassing at all. Why would it be wrong to use and focus the special abilities of certain people? We already do this all the time with forms of diversity that carry no stigmas. Neurodiversity also includes musical talent, for example. Nobody objects to using and focusing musical talents for a very specific purpose. Chess champions, Go players, gamers, mathematicians, visual artists, programmers, designers... We let them do what they're good at. And why wouldn't we?

To translate it into a practical example, most people appear to agree that it is pretty nuts that millions of us need to take off our shoes at airports and stand there holding a little baggie with small containers with any liquids we may want to take with us and that this is the response to two incidents that were actually dealt with effectively. These incidents were a plot discovered by British police in 2006 in which liquid explosives were going to be taken on board of airliners to the U.S. and Canada and the attempt by a British man to detonate a device hidden in his shoes on a

## Brain-based conditions 53

flight from France to the U.S. in 2001. (The story is that he had become radicalized when he spent time in prison for petty crimes and then went on to Afghanistan and Pakistan where he was trained by Al Qaeda.) The focus on shoes and liquids does not appear to accomplish anything practical and is as logical as banning all British people from flights and banning all flights from the U.K. because these incidents involved a Brit and planes taking off from Britain. I am willing to bet that people with NPD and/or psychopathy would have come up with much better solutions. (They'd only make us take off our shoes just to piss us off and poke fun at us.)

That is one of the good things about diversity. The variety! The cornucopia of skills and talents!

When I started diving into personality disorders, I realized that I had a friend with a narcissistic personality disorder. It is important to realize that there is a difference between having a disorder and being called a narcissist, by the way.

For decades, my friend and I got along just fine. Yes, she has hurt me on occasion, but other people have hurt me too and I too have hurt other people on occasion. It is part of life! In fact, I ended up hurting her badly, and that partly had to do with the way mental health professionals talk about people with NPD. I found that very confusing. It made me doubt myself. Was I wrong to trust and appreciate my friend the way I did? "Yes," was what the experts appeared to be saying. Was I truly that dense?

(As a result of my response, the friendship fell apart. It might not have happened if I had not been living in the U.K. at the time, as I might have been able to respond with more maturity – eh, less insecurity! – but that's immaterial now.)

It's highly ironic that members of the same professions (psychology and psychiatry) can also be very quick to dismiss people as delusional if those people look for support when they find themselves dealing with people with major personality disorders, but have no idea what they are dealing with.

Now, looking back, I can see that my friend actually had a great deal of trust towards me. She had said things to me that I didn't understand at all at the time. She had told me things about which she simply could have lied to me to make things easier for herself because it concerned things that I had no way of verifying. Instead, she made herself vulnerable to the risk of rejection and criticism. I feel ashamed about how I've let her down, but I also feel that I've let myself down. I knew my friend well enough to know that I should not expect the impossible from her. Heck, there are things that other people shouldn't expect from me either. I certainly knew very well that she sometimes responded in unusual ways. Now I understand why she may sometimes have felt joy when I encountered setbacks and why she couldn't always be happy for me when I achieved something but those occasions have been pretty rare.

It seems to me that people with NPD may often look for a kind of measuring standard that can tell them how they are doing. At the same time, they may very literally reflect back how you treat them because how you treat them tells them who they are. (And then they are either very happy or deeply disappointed.)

That I meanwhile have developed a better understanding of my friend's state of being probably means that I would now be able to handle any differences in opinion more intelligently than I have done on a few occasions in the now distant past.

Why should *she* have to tiptoe around *me* because I am neurotypical? I mean, we neurotypicals object to having to tiptoe around people who aren't neurotypical, object to having to take the difference into account and object to being more accommodating toward them, but we blindly expect them to do that around us. Why is that? Because there are more of "us" than of "them"?

Most of us neurotypicals probably barely know who we are and what drives us and what we need to thrive. We usually are barely aware of our emotions and how they control us. So we make it easy for some of the people in the long tail of brain-based diversity to push our buttons and the way we respond then puts a downward spiral in motion. Why can't we neurotypicals just keep standing on our own two feet instead? Why can't we choose to smile and keep breathing?

Maybe we also need more democracy with regard to neurodiversity.

Maybe we should keep this statement by Brenda Hale (a British judge who ended up heading the U.K's Supreme Court) in mind more often:

# Brain-based conditions

> *"The purpose of any human rights protection is to protect the rights of those whom the majority are unwilling to protect: democracy values everyone equally even if the majority do not."*

The full range of neurodiversity does not only run from for example extreme altruism on one end to psychopathy on the other. It does not only include states of being in which people suffer or cause suffering and states of being that are merely different. Synesthesia is a form of neurodiversity. Whether you have migraines or not can also be a form of neurodiversity. People also have these different states of being in different degrees. Neurodiversity is a multidimensional space, not a collection of either/or conditions.

At the moment, the neurodiversity we have still results in the marginalization of many people, who often have talents and abilities that neurotypicals lack. We may have a much greater need for those qualities in the future.

What I am doing right now, using a QWERTY keyboard to type words that leave room for misinterpretation and that are restricted to the English language, is a pretty limited form of communication. We will communicate very differently in the distant future. That could for example involve the transmission of images between our brains. Work is already underway that looks at brain activity and reads the images that our brains see. What if, for example, autistic people are much better at that and will need to lead the way, including teaching neurotypicals how to develop and use these skills?

Come to think of it, accepting diversity is partly also a matter of finding the right language to reach different people. Verbal communication certainly does have its limitations. Many artists communicate very differently. I remember when someone gave me the tip that "creative types" work and communicate very differently than "us computer-oriented or scientific types", shortly before I had a meeting with such a creative type. It is good to keep such things in mind and approach others with an open mind instead of with fixed expectations of how they should behave. (Again, I personally think that many English people are really simply plain crazy, however. I mean, that's blatantly obvious. ;-) Anyone can see that. Clearly.)

Perhaps the best illustration of why we have diversity and that it helps us deal with challenges is dissociative identity disorder (DID). This used to be called multiple personality disorder and is often confused with schizophrenia.

(I believed schizophrenia – about which I know next to nothing – to be completely different from DID until I saw a TED Talk by someone who had been diagnosed with a form of schizophrenia that sounded more like a form of DID to me. That brings back an echo of what I said about autism and psychopathy a few pages ago, so maybe *some* autism and *some* schizophrenia and *some* psychopathy are caused by external factors acting on very young developing brains, just like an arm that is broken over and over and over again. That provides a good analog for brain-based conditions. An open fracture does not mean that the arm is bad or that the person whose arm it is is bad, but that something happened to the arm. Here is the difficult part: By using a broken arm as an analogy I run the risk of seeming to suggest that neurodiversity needs to be "fixed". The problem with anything brain-based that has no physical consequences is not whether something may have been caused by external factors or not, the problem is society's lack of acceptance, the stigmatization and the lack of care and support when care and support are needed.)

Back to DID. Young children who are exposed to unbearable challenges can form multiple identities in their still-developing brains because the unique qualities of each of the individuals residing in their brains help them deal with the challenges they face. It's a form of solidarity. "If you're all alone, are dealing with horrible circumstances and have no one by your side, create your own support group" seems to be the strategy that such a developing brain applies.

The diversity that the brain can come up with in such circumstances is impressive and can include animals and even rocks. It's an immensely creative invention, born from a strong will to survive. People who live with such a condition aren't even mentally ill, though some of their identities can be. They do need to find a way to deal well with how their brain ticks and the first step toward that is understanding and acceptance. Sometimes, a form of healing may be possible that allows some of the identities to go to sleep or even "pass away". If there were no advantages in the wide range of diversity that DID displays, the human brain would not be using that the way it does. It wouldn't have come up

## Brain-based conditions

with that diversity. DID could have resulted in cloned personalities with different names, but the human brain does not see that as a solution. DID may hold major clues as to why (neuro)diversity exists. Neurodiversity has to contain major advantages for the human species, even though some of it surely will be simply the result of chance, like so many things.

By the way, the personality of each of us neurotypicals can also be much more in flux than we are usually willing to accept, or aware of. We don't like that idea. Most of us are terrified of the idea that our future self may have dementia, even though that future self may actually be a happier person with simpler interests than our current self. Where does that come from? The powerless we feel is one factor, and it's a major one, but the competitiveness of our western capitalist societies surely is another. What do I mean by that? Take depression. Some African regions appear to have much fewer cases of depression. That's because depression is seen as something that needs to be addressed by the community. Its existence is not denied, but it's not seen as an individual's "problem". (That may hold important cues for how us whities in the west. Yes, I am writing this book from the biased position of a white middle-aged woman in a western country. I know that I am overlooking many angles in this book because I am not aware of them and that is often because it's never been part of the cultures I've lived in.)

To come back to brain-based conditions, the common refusal to accept that other people's brain-based conditions genuinely exist, the refusal to accept that the people who have them cannot change themselves at will and cannot be blamed for having them goes hand in hand with a crazy fascination with certain brain-based disorders in a safely distanced manner (fiction in books and films) and a lot of fear-mongering.

That causes a gridlock. It leaves many people struggling on their own, often with everyone around them accusing them, vilifying them and disowning them or simply ignoring them. It probably causes a lot of understandable anger, frustration and powerlessness that has the capability of completely spinning out of control. I suspect that the lack of support for people with personality disorders and other mental health conditions can sometimes lead to the tragic excesses the public sometimes hears about. (Sadly, such tragic incidents are often instantly called terrorist attacks in some countries these days.)

**We need to talk about this**

Some people indeed do horrific things that are hard to understand. In the past decade, I have witnessed more cruelty than ever before and it provided me with some unexpected insights. This cruelty came from people in my surroundings and was deliberately aimed at me, to spite me. The situation's gone on for over a decade now and appears to classify as so-called sadistic stalking. It's a complicated and challenging (taxing) situation that's had serious consequences for my life and also for my physical health, but not necessarily a hopeless one. I am trying to make it work by creating synergy and by learning from it as much as I can. I am hoping to extend what I am learning to be able to help others in similar situations. Communication – mismatches in communication style – seems to play a major role in these situations and in neurodiversity in general.

I learned an important lesson from it. When you are exposed to a lot of cruelty, and for a long time, you become on edge, nervous about the next bad thing that is going to happen. For a while, I was permanently anxious in anticipation of what might be next. This is very unhealthy for the body. I suspect that this is why the fear and disgust response can begin to disappear after a while. I observed that my own response to repeatedly seeing cruelty began to change. I found that a very worrisome development and I made a successful effort to rein it in and stop it. I later learned that this may be a response from the endocrine system to shield the body against harmful effects of prolonged high levels of stress.

It taught me something about how sadistic traits may come about in young children who suffer horrific abuse again and again and again or why long-term kidnapping victims sometimes go on to do horrible things. Their response becomes blunted and then it starts to change. This change is not a choice. What I noticed in me happened beyond my control and it horrified me, frankly. As an adult with many other experiences and with well-functioning "brakes" in your mind, you can notice something like this in yourself – and intervene, however. Very young children who have never experienced anything else but cruelty cannot do that. So such children may either develop DID to keep themselves whole or develop serious personality disorders with severe sadistic traits. (People who don't have a strong psychological core may be more susceptible to this too.)

Unfortunately, any kind of "mental health" condition – even when it is merely temporary just like many physical conditions – tends to burden

## Brain-based conditions 59

people with a lasting stigma. Why? Why is it still much more accepted to be in a hospital with appendicitis or meningitis than because of a suicide attempt or a psychotic episode? It makes it so much harder for people to get the support they need when they need it.

There may be a solution that can help turn a lot of this around, both the stigma and the refusal to accept the reality of brain-based conditions, the refusal to accept the fact that people can have different brain structures and may genuinely not be able to control their behavior. (Notably, autistic children are often labeled spoiled or ill-behaved or naughty. Their parents are judged, too.)

Research has found that it can help toward the acceptance of so-called mental health conditions to translate them into visual information. Show people a brain scan of the person in their surroundings who is "not well in the head" and let them see how it deviates from a neurotypical brain's scan. If the blood chemistry differs, show them that, in a colorful graph. It also makes acceptance easier for the people who have such brain-based conditions.

The visualization of the condition is the "broken arm" that tells other people that there really is something going on and that there is good reason to be mindful of the "arm" and avoid bumping into it. It helps people see that it really makes no sense to blame the person for the mental condition that he or she never asked for. It reveals that the person isn't merely "behaving badly all the time" and is not refusing to "grow up".

I would like to see this go further. In Britain, several lengthy reports, including by the police's own watchdog, have found that police forces are failing massively in how they deal with reports of stalking. In all the assessed cases, the police officers involved let people down. This kind of failure leads to ruined lives, both among the stalking targets and among the stalkers. (If there is almost no support for victims, even in more serious cases of stalking, then how much support, do you reckon, is there for people who engage in stalking behaviors, for whom the threshold to seek support is much higher?) It sometimes also leads to injuries and deaths that could have been avoided. This calls for a very different, much more efficient approach that would free up regular police officers to focus more on the jobs they are supposed to do instead of having to deal with topics most officers are not trained for and are not equipped for.

For starters, police officers are not in any position to be able to assess someone's state of mind or mental health situation. At the moment, police officers still play an important role in caring for people with brain-based health conditions, however. Would you want police officers to operate on your heart or assess whether you may have breast cancer? If not, then why are we letting police officers play the lead role in so many situations that involve brain-based conditions?

Seven years ago, organizations in the Netherlands decided that people who are "confused", as the Dutch call it ("verward" or "in de war"), should no longer be allowed to land in police cells if no crime had been committed (the latter is, of course, also a matter for debate). Such people would no longer be put in handcuffs and bundled into police cars but transported in "psycholances". Here we go again. I find this an offensive term because of its association with the word "psycho", which has so many negative connotations (also in Dutch). It is easy enough to give such vehicles a much more neutral name like "hersenambulance" or "hersenzorg" ("brain ambulance" or "brain care") or even "GGZ ambulance" ("mental healthcare ambulance").

Despite this, 75% of these patients were transported in Dutch police vehicles instead of ambulances in 2019. That year, there were over 96,000 reports about "confused people" in the country; around 2,300 people still ended up in a cell at a police station. The 2019 number of reports was twice the number of reports made in 2011. This has to do with the dismantling of care for people with brain-related conditions in the Netherlands. In the city of Rotterdam, 20% of those hospital beds were lost in 2012 alone; by the end of 2020, there will have been a decline of 33%.

In 2017, Rotterdam police officers were also the ones who tasered a naked patient who was already in solitary confinement at a hospital. They tasered him more than thirty times, in so-called pain compliance mode and even on the soles of his feet, for reasons that remain utterly unclear. Amnesty International was appalled, along with many other organizations. The hospital regretted what had happened and allegedly filed a complaint about the tasering. When Dutch officers are called to a mental health hospital, they take over all responsibility. Can it get any crazier than that? Police officers are never called to the hospital when a

## Brain-based conditions 61

patient throws a clot during a surgery or is coming out of a coma, so why should police be called to a hospital and take over responsibility for a patient who has a brain-based condition?

Police forces in the Netherlands have been asking for more trained mental health professionals and more support for people with brain-based health conditions who live in the community. They have signaled that police officers are simply not equipped to assess someone's health condition and they don't want to have to play doctor any longer. I haven't heard similar calls for more medical staff involvement in communities from police forces in the U.K. yet (but I may simply have missed them). In Rotterdam, persons who are confused (including people with, for example, dementia) currently cause at least one fire per week.

Police officers generally assess someone's mental health and level of potential danger on the basis of how obedient and compliant someone is in response to orders given by police officers. Asserting one's rights or simply not responding – also for example by deaf people or because someone does not want to undress in front of male police officers or because the person is in his or her own home or yard and sees no reason to comply with nonsensical orders barked by a stranger who may not even be wearing a police uniform – can quickly get someone considered a "problem case", notably if you are of a certain age or have a certain skin tone. But if you act in a docile robot-like manner and do as told, you are considered fine. That's utterly nuts.

The Netherlands was supposed to get a new national phone number to call with regard to "people who are confused", but it has not materialized yet. The Dutch continue to have to call the police unless they live in an area that has organized its own regional phone number.

Police should not have to play a role in health care. I would not want to take my car to the butcher or buy bread from a garbage collection van. So why do police officers continue to have to play the role of medical professionals? It means that in practice, police officers are perhaps the biggest reinforcers of mental health stigma. For starters, having to call the police for someone with a brain-based health condition suggests that the person has done something wrong and deserves to be punished.

To sum it up, all states of being have advantages and disadvantages and this also goes for brain-based diversity. To a large degree, it is a matter of needing greater equality (or "equity", as some people call it, to distinguish it from "treating everyone the same"). When we talk about equality and equal opportunities, opponents often reject this as a ridiculous concept. The short story "Harrison Bergeron" by Kurt Vonnegut illustrates very well what they mean. It paints a world in which the sports practice of handicapping is applied to humans. The size and nature of the added handicap clearly reveal the characteristics of the person underneath the mask and costume.

That is not at all what the concept of "equal opportunities" is about. It is about not discriminating between different people who can do something equally well. It is about not making life more difficult for some people than for others. It is about ensuring everyone gets food, shelter and medical care and all the other human rights, including the right to live and to live one's life freely. It is about not holding some people back and encouraging others, about allowing everyone room to thrive, to flourish. It is about enablement and empowerment.

It is about allowing Nicolas Joncour to go to school instead of sticking him in a psychiatric institution, beating him, or chaining him to his bed or to a wall. He isn't even mentally unwell. His brain works fine, but it works differently. He communicates differently. Not being allowed to use your magnificent brain and being locked up, deprived of experiences, is enough to drive most people around the bend and scar them for life. Depriving children of meaningful communications impacts how their brains develop.

# 7. Lives not worth living

*"Life is not worth living if I cannot have pasta or bread again."*

– Monica Seles

I wanted to know whether it was possible to come up with a universally applicable guideline for the new eugenics that respects diversity and prevents harm as much as possible. Such a guideline would have to be amended eventually, but we need a course and a compass that we can use right now.

To create generally applicable regulations that don't collapse at the first legal challenge, we first need to come up with generally applicable definitions. Within the context of consumer eugenics (tinkering with our offspring, germline modifications), we must act primarily in the interest of the child and we must prevent any harm to the child (and that includes the resulting adult).

But what constitutes harm within this context?

First of all, we have this principle:

**Allowing someone to be created does not harm that person.**

This is a generally accepted view that I agree with, even though there are groups of people who believe that it is wrong to have children, for various reasons.

But if I accept that for example a hearing child and a deaf child are equally valuable, I run into the problem that if a hearing child is injured in such a way that the child loses his or her hearing, we do consider that harm. This also applies when it concerns adults and the laws in most countries agree with this view. Companies ensure the safety of their employees, for example, for that reason.

That forces me to ask myself whether it constitutes harm to allow a child to be born without hearing (or to be born with a condition that will eventually render it deaf).

If I explore that, then the following becomes clear:

We consider it harm when someone else changes us against our wishes, particularly with regard to physical changes.

We seem to be less clear on psychological changes, and that is because they are much harder to identify and quantify. We don't start lawsuits against bad schools and bad teachers when they have hampered or changed our children in a way that good schools and good teachers don't – even though the former can also mar a child for life. To a large degree, we still rely on the presence of a physical component to consider something harmful enough.

We don't generally think that a surgeon harms a person if that person decides to undergo cosmetic surgery for purely aesthetic reasons, but would consider it harm if this were to happen against the person's wishes. (There can of course also be harm if the surgeon is professionally negligent in the sense of using the wrong sutures or other errors, but that is not the context we're talking about here.)

So the crux appears to be this:

**We should not change another person (physically) if that change isn't that person's explicit wish.**

(The right to integrity of the body also plays a role here.)

A child who doesn't exist yet can neither express nor have wishes yet, which is why I then have to make the following decision:

**We should assume that any change we would carry out to that child is not based on that child's wishes but against its wishes.**

That is a potentially problematic conclusion.

Should this then also for example include PGD, as PGD itself can do damage? No, because actions to detect and identify conditions or diseases are excluded from what constitutes harm, as they are – or should be – applied to prevent harm, for example, to make it possible to treat a baby from birth as opposed to letting the parents take the baby home, only to have it diagnosed later with a condition that could have been treated from the start, which might have prevented a lot of pain. Techniques like PGD would also help detect conditions that lead to lives not worth living (which I also still need to define, but I'll come to that).

On the other hand, genetic changes accomplished by techniques such as

CRISPR should be included (that is, considered harm), unless they are done to enable lives that would otherwise not be possible and/or treat developing health problems.

(Remember that I am looking for a guideline that we can use right now. Such a guideline, if adopted, can and very likely will have to be adapted later. By then, we will have a lot more experience with technologies like CRISPR and we'll have gained a lot more insight. This is theoretical doodling. You can even call it wishful thinking if you want.)

Generally speaking, however, we also have to take this into account:

**Until a child reaches majority, the parents are required to make decisions for the child and in the child's best interest.**

Is there a potential conflict here, between not doing something against someone else's wishes, the inability of the very young to have and express wishes of their own hence the parents needing to act on their behalf? I need to explore this further.

It is acceptable to most people – though not everyone, mostly on religious grounds – that parents ensure that medical intervention takes place when this is required to save a child's life. If a healthy child contracts a disease or suffers an injury that without medical intervention would result in a so-called diminishment (or death), the latter also clearly counts as a change that would take place against the child's wishes whereas the medical treatment would be according to its wishes. No child wants to have appendicitis, for example, and not be treated for it and it is also very unlikely that a hearing or seeing child would genuinely want to be deaf or blind. So there does not seem to be a conflict here. (That said, in a very noisy environment, being deaf would be a blessing.)

Yes, a child that wants its ears pierced may ask for this as a result of peer pressure, but it is still a wish that comes from the child. It is akin to an adult asking for cosmetic surgery for purely aesthetic reasons. That too is the result of some form of societal pressure. No one should force a child to have its ears pierced; that would be harm. Also, a parent can stop a child from having its ears or nose pierced based on the argument that the child is too young to be able to make such decisions and the procedure is not a medical necessity. There definitely seems to be no conflict here either.

So it looks like this definition of harm holds up and would not get in the way of parental duties to existing children (children that have been born and are alive, as opposed to children that do not exist yet).

Changes implemented not explicitly according to our wishes must be seen as occurring against our wishes, and constitute harm. (Note that this would also apply to male circumcision and female genital mutilation.)

**So, in principle, any changes carried out to a child who doesn't exist yet must be assumed to be against that child's explicit wishes, hence constitute harm, unless that change would enable a life that would otherwise either not be worth living or not even possible.**

Now I have a basis that I can work with.

I now also can say the following (but keep in mind that I still need to define what a life not worth living is).

**We cause harm if we create a child who will have a life not worth living if we are able to prevent that.**

However, a child born into such a life without the parents' prior awareness that the child would have that kind of life is not harmed by the parents because the parents weren't in a position to prevent this life on the basis of the knowledge they had. (This is important.)

Note that this definition also implies that if we can remedy the situation, for example through the use of CRISPR or an abortion, we should.

But what is a life not worth living?

Most people probably see "a life not worth living" in terms of physical pain and of increasing, terrible suffering that will only lead to the child's death. The parents and other persons in the child's surroundings may gain something from the experience and possibly become more compassionate as a result, but the child gains absolutely nothing from the experience. On the contrary, it only suffers.

At this point in history, it is not possible to say how much pain the child suffers, or whether it is even aware of the pain. We don't know.

We can't leave "a life not worth living" undefined, however. It would leave the door open for people acting on the basis of personal opinions or feelings that have little to do with the resulting child's welfare. It could

# Lives not worth living

also mean that every case would have to be looked at individually, which would soon cease to be practical. So we need a definition that we can apply to every case, in principle.

I need a basis for defining what makes a life worth living.

For that, I use the following principle:

**Every human being has the right to a life in dignity.**

This is the so-called principle of humanity. (See the 2003 working paper by Buchanan-Smith or the course "Humanitarian response to conflict and disaster" by the Harvard Humanitarian Initiative and Harvard Center for Health and Human Rights.)

We probably agree on this principle of humanity worldwide, no matter where we are from or what our religious background is. So this can offer the first step toward a definition of "a life not worth living".

But... what is dignity?

As it turns out, it is not possible to decide what constitutes dignity for someone else. We can only define it for ourselves. Consider that nudity equals a lack of dignity for many people, but not at all for many other people. Being too ill to eat and use the bathroom without assistance can constitute an unbearable lack of dignity for one person but be acceptable to someone else. Being unable to breathe and needing a ventilator may be where the latter person draws the line, while someone else may still find that acceptable but would, on the other hand, like to avoid being in a coma or some other form of vegetative state for, say, more than a month.

These physical forms of loss of dignity are not the only ones imaginable. Alzheimer's, for example, can cause a loss of dignity too, even though it has its basis in physical developments in the brain. Almost all of us would likely want to avoid getting Alzheimer's disease. However, one reason for excessive alcohol consumption is the loss of awareness it results in and you can probably see drunkenness as akin to temporary Alzheimer's. Just like we can adapt to natural physical changes, we could also decide now that we would accept natural changes to our future selves, such as Alzheimer's, and would adjust our expectations accordingly. The person who you are today may not be the person who you will be twenty years from now. But I digress.

Dignity clearly is a personal concept. It is the result of cultural and religious influences and one's personal preferences and experiences.

The examples I just gave, of being on a ventilator and so on, are western and contemporary, but that does not matter. The principle of dignity itself, however, will very likely hold for a long time, even if our views change of what is acceptable and what not.

This takes me to the next step.

**To be able to decide whether we are living a life in dignity or not, we have to be able to make decisions.**

So now we have the following:

- To allow a human being to come into the world does not constitute harm to that human being.

- To allow a human being to come into the world constitutes harm if that human being will have a life not worth living, if this was known in advance and if it was possible to prevent that.

- To implement physical changes (including genetic changes) against a person's explicit wishes constitutes harm.

- As unborn children are not yet able to express wishes, any changes (including genetic changes) carried out to unborn children must be seen as being against the explicit wishes of those children, with the exception of a change that would enable the child to come into the world (meaning that without the change, the pre-embryo or embryo would not be viable) or heal, the way we would also try to heal appendicitis or a potentially fatal yet fixable heart problem.

- All humans have a right to a life with dignity (the principle of humanity).

- It is not possible to define dignity for another person.

- To be able to decide whether a person has a life with dignity, that person has to be able to make and communicate decisions, with or without explicit assistance.

- A person gains the right to make his or her own decisions at majority (full age, coming of age). In many countries, this is the age of 18 years. This is therefore a logical age to attach to this guideline (and attaching a fixed age limit to my non-discrimination guideline for embryos helps rule out arbitrariness).

With the above, we can create a workable definition of "a life not worth living".

**A life not worth living is a life that has at least a 95% probability of not making it to the age of 18 or that has at least a 95% probability of the person not being able to make and communicate his or her own decisions at that age, even with assistance.**

I feel that it is necessary to point out that this does not represent my personal preference. I am repulsed by the idea of declaring that someone who passes away at age 4 or 9 or 15 does not have a life worth living. I came up with this definition because it seems to work very well in practice and that means that it contains little risk of arbitrariness or corruption. This definition also does appear to diminish harm as much as possible while not promoting discrimination or prejudice, hence respecting diversity.

It holds up for severe psychopathy as well. If a gene, allele or genetic combination is identified that predicts a 95% likelihood that someone will engage in arson, torture of animals and so on without there being a cure or treatment to prevent this from happening, then such persons would also fall within the category of persons who are unable to make their own decisions at the age of majority. They would make their decisions on the basis of harm to others and seek to harm, instead of avoiding it. This means that such a person would have a life not worth living, clearly also for his or her own sake. This would likely only pertain to rare cases, in practice.

The ability to make decisions is useless without being able to communicate them. Appropriate assistance should be able to achieve that communication if needed, and we have to be diligent in this respect. Persons who require assistance with the actual decision-making should have that assistance. Most of us enjoy some kind of assistance in our decision-making, regardless of whether we are aware of it.

### Identity, legal persons and rights

Some bioethicists strongly object to the treatment of pre-embryos and embryos (as well as fetuses) as if they aren't humans. When does a person begin and when do his or her rights begin? Within the context of liability of the parents in cases of intentional "diminishment" (selection of pre-embryos with a certain trait such as deafness), some scholars have mentioned identity. That raises very complicated questions for which there are no answers. At what point can we say that we have changed someone's identity? At what point does someone's identity begin? Nobody knows. Identity is partly, and maybe even mostly, formed after birth, and so that discussion only seems to lead further astray instead of providing more clarity.

But both that approach and mine run into the same problem: Can someone who does not exist yet – a pre-embryo or even a not yet existing embryo – be seen as a person, and therefore be assigned rights?

If not, then how can there be harm if, for example, we were to carry out genetic changes to an embryo, under the assumption that this would be against the future child's wishes? (I mean this within the context of the law, not morally speaking.) If yes, then how can we legally allow any form of abortion of embryos of up to 24 weeks and not consider it murder?

We, therefore, seem to have a need for a new international category of legal personhood. If a business can be a person and a river and a mountain in New Zealand can be legal persons, then surely it is also possible to have a separate category of legal personhood for pre-embryos and embryos or fetuses up to 24 weeks. (An embryo is generally considered a fetus when it is at least 10 weeks old, so I understand, but in this book, I have mostly used the currently often used time limit of 24 weeks, the point up to which abortion is commonly allowed, although this point is not set in stone.)

Cell clusters in those stages would not have a legal right to life yet (so this would therefore not clash with existing abortion rights), but they should have the right not be discriminated against on the basis of the characteristics of the eventually resulting person (child) unless those characteristics would give the child a life not worth living. This safeguards basic human rights concepts like respect and dignity as well as the principle of unconditional love as the basis for good parenthood

## Lives not worth living

and inclusive solidarity in society.

This may be a stretch for many and take some getting used to.

For the time being, such cell clusters should also have the right not be interfered with in a way that would constitute harm if similar actions were carried out on a newborn. We wouldn't want to apply CRISPR to a newborn so that its eye color would match the home furnishings better, so we shouldn't do it to gametes or pre-embryos either.

A pre-embryo that does not yet exist, of course, does not have any rights and cannot be harmed. You could perceive sperm and egg selection based on their characteristics as a human rights violation, but the problem with that is that a human who never comes into existence doesn't have any rights. Here too, however, we can apply the principle of non-discrimination to sperm and egg selection. Sperm and egg selection should take place "blindfolded" (which is what I also argue for abortion). Lives not worth living should be the only exceptions and conditions such as genetic deafness or dwarfism do not fall into that category of lives not worth living.

**We need to talk about this**

## 8. A guideline for the new eugenics

*"I know we can't abolish prejudice through laws, but we can set up guidelines for our actions by legislation."*

– Belva Lockwood

As discussed in earlier chapters in this book, enhancing or designing our offspring does not provide guarantees for our offspring's wellbeing or even competitiveness at this point (with the limited knowledge that we currently have).

And as I have also made clear in the previous chapters, I believe that for the time being, we should restrict ourselves, for the following reasons.

- At this point, we are unable to predict the effects of allowing an unbridled practice of personal or mandatory eugenics on the human species. We have made many mistakes in the past when we blindly applied what we thought of as technological advances without being able to see their future deleterious effects.
- Perceived impairments are often hindrances created by society.
- Human variations that some people may currently think of as less valuable (less competitive or less worth having around) may become much more valuable in the future. We can't assess what we don't know yet.
- There is a potential for harm to the resulting child if the child does not meet its parents' expectations, for whatever reasons.

Here is what I propose for the practices of personal (and mandatory) eugenics:

**Only allow selection that selects against children who have at least a 95% probability of not making it to their 18th birthday or who have at least a 95% probability of not being able to make their own decisions at that age, with or without assistance.**

I am aware that some countries already have an accepted practice that goes beyond what I propose.

The medical profession can give us the statistical probabilities for whether or not a child will be able to make its own decisions at the age of 18 (age of majority, coming of age), given it has a certain genetic condition. There is no such thing as 100% certainty in most of these cases. All we need is a good enough certainty, something that we can work with (also in the courts). We can work this out in such a way that we don't need to be concerned about the validity of the statistics (bias). We could, for example, ask all countries to supply their individual assessments and use the average.

Gut feelings against this type of reasoning can be very strong, such as the impression that this way of thinking diminishes the value of some lives, no matter how short. I have those feelings too. This is not necessarily a problem, however. Parents who feel very strongly about this are unlikely to select against such a baby and are also highly unlikely to sue a state to get what they want. The courts only need to know how to deal with cases that are brought before them. Cases that do not show up in the courts solve themselves.

I also have some doubts about how people will determine whether someone can make his or her own decisions. If you consider that for a very long time, we've thought that other animals had no cognitive abilities and were not able to feel emotions, hence were not able to make conscious decisions either…

At this point, I don't think we should criminalize the decision to accept a life, but this may of course change in the future. By that, I mean that we may have to decide that an embryo or pre-embryo that will result in a baby with Lesch-Nyhan syndrome must not be implanted and that embryos or fetuses that test positive for such conditions must be aborted.

Thus, the implantation of for example an embryo that would lead to genetic deafness would be allowed and would not be a condition that we would test for as a basis for deselection. I think we should carry out much more extensive tests at birth (many of which we currently don't do yet, also for certain infections) so that we can treat children from birth and not, for example, be forced to diagnose them at 1, 2 or 5 years old when a lack of a certain protein has already done a lot of damage to the child's body (and mind). Testing at birth including brain imaging, if possible, should also be carried out for personality disorders and other conditions that are considered to be of a mental nature, and then followed up by the provision of support just like we also support persons with physical conditions. Brain scans would also detect irregularities such as neuroblastomas.

If the regulations state that discriminatory selection of eggs, sperm and pre-embryos is not allowed unless it would prevent a life not worth living as I have defined here, we would have a great deal more clarity than we seem to have now.

The principle of what constitutes a life not worth living as I have defined it here seems to hold up well in practice. Some examples are Tay-Sachs disease, Lesch-Nyhan syndrome, Leigh syndrome, types of severe combined immunodeficiency (SCID) and (some cases of) mitochondrial DNA depletion syndrome. (Keep in mind that this should also go hand in hand with applying techniques like CRISPR first to enable these lives and remedy lives not worth living.)

From what I've written in this booklet, it automatically follows that mitochondrial replacement therapy (MRT) – colloquially known as the creation of three-parent babies – should be allowed (technical and practical issues aside) because it would enable the creation of lives that wouldn't be possible without MRT. (I feel that it is not my place to tell a family unable to create offspring without ART to adopt an orphan.) This may change in the future, possibly leading to more snowbabies. As we cannot possibly know the long-term effects of the application of such techniques, MRT should only be used as a last resort. Britain and Mexico are examples of countries that allow the clinical application of MRT.

I am not saying that this guideline should always remain in place. A common response to the previous two versions of this book was that people let me know "I don't agree with you" without specifying what they meant, and I suspect it had to do with this guideline. I am not saying that we need to keep proceeding this way, but that we should do this for the time being. It would allow us to gain more knowledge and, very importantly, limit any harm that we do while we explore the applicability of technologies like CRISPR. Once we have enough experience, we can slowly take it forward.

**We need to talk about this**

Future societies will be different, just like I grew up without a mobile phone and tablet while many of today's children have at least a mobile phone. Whatever I prefer personally should play no role. What is good for the human species should play a role (and this has to include concern for other species; see also Chapter 9). I do not think that relocating to Mars is a good option if we don't take the time to learn and be able to apply the lessons that we are taught on this planet. We can't keep wrecking planets and moving to different planets endlessly.

**An exercise**

To get an idea of the current practice, let's take a look at what the U.K.'s Human Fertilisation and Embryology Authority (HFEA) does. It uses a growing list that currently contains about 400 conditions that pre-embryos can be tested against, but this means that couples must use IVF. In 2005, the HFEA issued the consultation "Choices & Boundaries: Should people be able to select embryos free from an inherited susceptibility to cancer?" "We want to hear the views of patients, carers and representatives of affected families, staff in treatment centres, disability groups, parliamentarians, academics and the wider public about the use of PGD for these types of conditions," the Chair of HFEA stated in the introduction.

That consultation contained the following questions (see hereafter). If you didn't take part in it, how would you have answered these questions? Do you think that embryos who have a high breast cancer probability should not be allowed to develop into babies and grow into adults? Why, or why not? Do we have the right to withhold life from such an embryo? What about the embryo that would be allowed to be born instead if the embryo with the high breast cancer chance is discarded? Should that embryo be given to other parents, perhaps? In December 2017, a few days before Christmas, an American woman gave birth to a baby whose embryo was frozen in 1992. She felt that that baby would be as good as any other baby, even though it is not genetically related to her. (Such children are called snowbabies.)

- Question 1: We are interested to find out how you feel about using PGD to test for lower penetrance conditions such as inherited breast cancer. To help put your views about this in context, it is important to understand how you feel about PGD for fully penetrant conditions such as cystic fibrosis or haemophilia. Do you agree with the use of PGD in general. For example, for fully penetrant conditions that are present in the child?

- Question 2: The HFEA guidance to PGD centres states that PGD should only be available where there is significant risk of a serious genetic condition. Given the lower penetrance, later age of onset and potential treatability of inherited cancer conditions, do you consider them to be serious genetic conditions?

- Question 3: The HFEA guidance to PGD centres states that PGD should only be available where there is significant risk of a serious genetic condition. Does the penetrance of the condition affect whether or not you consider it to confer a significant risk? In your opinion what would be the lowest penetrance – in percentage terms – that would confer significant risk?

- Question 4: The HFEA guidance to PGD centres states that the views of the people seeking treatment should be taken into account when considering whether to offer PGD. There needs to be a balance between the views of those people who would seek to use PGD to avoid passing on a condition and the views of wider society that may have ethical concerns about them doing so. In your opinion, how much emphasis should be placed on the views of those people seeking treatment?

- Question 5: The HFEA guidance to PGD centres states that the use of PGD should be consistent with current practice in prenatal diagnosis. Do you agree, with respect to lower-penetrance conditions, that the availability of PGD should be determined by current practice in prenatal diagnosis?

- Question 6: The HFEA wants to know where you feel the boundaries for the use of PGD lie. Considering penetrance, age of onset and treatability, what type of condition do you think should never be tested for in embryos using PGD?

The Scottish Council on Human Bioethics spoke out very clearly. Among other things, it said the following:

"Given that many respected organisations, and various national legislations, consider the early embryo to be due full protection as a human being, the SCHB regrets that U.K. legislation regards the early embryo as so readily dispensable."

It also wrote:

"the practice of PGD is fundamentally flawed as it fails to recognise the true nature of, and hence undervalues, human embryos. Following the creation of the embryo, when the genetic composition of the individual is determined, the development of this embryo is a continuous process right through to adulthood. Any attempt to demarcate a point in this process, before which an embryo should be considered a person, is arbitrary. In the absence of clear evidence to the contrary, the precautionary principle dictates that even the earliest embryo should be accorded full protection as a human being."

On 21 January 2013, HFEA responded to the question of whether HFEA had, prior to 2008, received a PGD application to select in favor of a disability. The answer was negative (F-2013-00009 - PGD applications in favour of disability).

I believe that the advent of artificial wombs (uteruses) will provide a way out of the dilemma that currently still pitches so many people and institutions against each other based on the opposing views they have on the rights of embryos. When abortion ceases to be required or desirable in certain circumstances as offspring are created in labs and grown in artificial wombs, procreation becomes a chosen and parenting perhaps an assigned privilege, today's reasons to discard embryos will have disappeared. It will be possible much sooner before it will become mainstream, however. On Twitter, Hank Greely (Stanford) said that it will likely take 50 to 100 years. I think it may begin to happen sooner.

## Implications for wrongful conception, wrongful birth and wrongful life cases

Three kinds of lawsuits are particularly relevant for what I propose. Wrongful conception and pregnancy, wrongful birth, and wrongful life cases are currently all based on the idea of negligence on the part of labs, hospitals or medical professionals.

## A guideline for the new eugenics

Wrongful pregnancy or wrongful conception cases imply that the parents who bring such a case didn't want a child. Any child. Think of unsuccessful voluntary sterilization as an example. This does not clash with what I propose. There is no element of discrimination here.

Wrongful birth cases are lawsuits by parents who have had a child with a significant disability or impairment. These cases can have an element of discrimination. These are cases against, for example, doctors who should have informed the parents about a medical condition in the (pre)embryo or fetus, the parents claiming that in that event, they would have opted for abortion. Usually, the parents claim damages due to psychological upset and financial damages related to extra costs involved in caring for the child. In practice, these claims usually contain an element of medical malpractice (negligence), an element of the need to find financing for a child's care or both.

As Ronen Perry pointed out in his 2008 paper, in these cases (as well as in wrongful life claims), the medical professionals (or labs) involved tended to have provided reassurances, rather than having for example amputated the wrong leg or, as happened in Britain recently, having amputated breasts that did not need to be removed. Of course, one of the problems medical professionals face is that the public wants to receive a 100% guarantee from them, which is impossible. That, however, usually isn't at the heart of the matter here. Rather than having provided reassurances too lavishly, labs or medical professionals tend to have messed up in these cases (mixed up samples, sent the wrong results, omitted to do a test or carried out a test incorrectly, etc). Understandably, parents may end up feeling badly wronged, and it is also understandable that parents seek redress through the courts rather than through the medical regulatory authorities. However, there is also always the question of how these parents would have responded if the condition of their child had been the result of a traffic accident or a fall down the stairs at the age of 1.

In 2014, Mpaate Owagage published a clear analysis of the developments with regard to wrongful life cases. "A wrongful life claim", he wrote, "is one brought for or on behalf of a usually extremely disabled plaintiff who claims recompense on the basis that but for the defendant's negligence, they would not have existed at all." When courts do award damages, these cases essentially become wrongful birth cases, except that the damages are awarded to the claimant (plaintiff) and not to the claimant's parent(s), thereby essentially safeguarding the claimant's care. Ivo Giesen analyzed the ins and outs in an article published in 2012 and held that "most notably the cultural background and/or the legal policy reasons within a certain tort law/medical liability law system" decide the issue in practice.

Wrongful life cases are problematic. They are started by or on behalf of a child or resulting adult. They tend to hinge on three factors. The first one is the question of whether the defendant had a duty of care toward the claimant. If so, the second question is whether this duty has been breached by the defendant and, third, whether this resulted in demonstrable damages for the claimant (for which damages may be awarded).

There are two different types of wrongful life cases, as well as two different legal approaches (see article by Owagage), but these two do not fully overlap. The difference in the cases rests on the principle of harm as I have identified it in this book, namely the occurrence of a physical change that can easily be assumed to occur against a person's will.

In cases in which the child has for example Tay-Sachs disease or any other genetic condition, the child has this condition irrespective of what a physician, hospital or lab did. Nobody caused this condition. The condition is not the result of an action (other than the creation of the zygote from which the child developed). (This will change in the future when a duty may develop to carry out techniques like CRISPR on such an embryo, but it will change in the opposite way.) So it cannot be said that the defendant caused any damage to the claimant. This becomes muddled when we consider the creation of a zygote in the lab, but in that case, why not sue the parents too, as they are primarily responsible for the child's existence? But even for such cases, the world seems to be growing toward the consensus that to be alive does not constitute damage in itself.

In cases in which the child's mother for example had rubella during early pregnancy, however, physical changes did occur. These changes would not have occurred if rubella had not been present. At first, this seems significant, but in these cases too, all logic leads back to one overriding question, namely whether the child would have been better off if it had not existed. This could have allowed a different child to exist

# A guideline for the new eugenics 81

that would not have been affected by, for example, rubella, but this is irrelevant.

However, in these cases, the claimants "do not contend that the defendant caused the deformity", Owagage pointed out in his analysis. The claimants pose that the defendant was negligent in making information available to the parents.

To understand the dilemma, it is helpful to compare the situation with that of a five-year-old child being hit in traffic by a drunk driver. Is the driver's liability greater when the child ends up paralyzed relative to when the child dies? Can the child (or the parents) sue the driver because the driver did not kill the child, but paralyzed the child instead? No.

(It is hard to find an exact parallel among cases with five-year-olds, with similar relationships between professionals, child and parents as in wrongful life cases. That said, there is a duty of care toward the child on the side of the driver, and road traffic accidents too are mainly negligence cases. So the comparison seems a valuable exercise.)

Is a child better off when it falls down the stairs and dies than when it falls down the stairs and becomes a paraplegic?

Now consider the case in which both parents are blind and deaf and have just moved to a different neighborhood. Can the professional who sold them the house be held negligent if he or she has failed to inform the parents that a busy road runs past the property if the child subsequently walks into traffic and gets hit by a car? The real estate professional was in possession of vital information that the parents did not have. Had they had that information, the parents might have had a better gate installed, so that the accident would not have occurred that affected the life of the child. But would the child (or the parents) sue the real estate professional because the child didn't die?

Such a hypothetical case seems very relevant with respect to the wrongful life scenario, particularly if the real estate professional provided a statement in writing that the house was sound, whereas someone else took photos at the time that clearly show that it wasn't. (We have to ignore that there may be an element of ill will in this example.)

If a house has a brick chimney that is about to fall off, the real estate agent fails to mention this to the blind parents, and their child is injured by the falling bricks from the chimney, that would be like a health professional withholding information from a pregnant woman as a result of which the fetus is affected by rubella. This child, however, would not sue the real estate professional because it is still alive, but the child could bring an action for the damage done by the falling chimney.

Then it begins to look like the distinction between the two different kinds of wrongful life cases is important. It also becomes clear that being alive in itself is clearly not considered "damage" as the child would not take the driver or real estate professional to court because it is still alive.

It then becomes clear that some wrongful life cases do seem to have a real basis, whereas others don't.

In the cases of genetic conditions, when the mother claims that she would have terminated the pregnancy had she had the correct information, the child cannot claim that it would have been better to be dead (with the exception of a life "not worth living").

If you want to draw a parallel with non-existing versus existing or a different child existing instead, you could consider the fact that one child may get hit by a car while a child standing at a distance of 1 meter does not. Someone who gets hit by a car cannot claim that if he or she had stood in another person's position, the car might not have hit anyone. Someone who does not get hit by the car cannot bring a lawsuit against the driver, claiming that the driver hit the wrong person. Who gets hit by a car or not, that is almost always a similarly philosophical question as occurs when courts are asked to consider wrongful life cases involving genetic conditions. It's almost like curved space-time.

It is impossible to know whether the car might have swerved or spun out of control differently if the person had stood in a different position or if the sun had been shining or the sun had not been shining.

In wrongful life cases in which the mother contracted rubella, it makes more sense for the child to sue the mother than the physician, but not for the fact that the child or resulting person exists but for the fact that a physical change was caused against the child's explicit will. This, however, is currently not a reasonable course of action. A mother has no control over whether someone who for example happens to be on the same train happens to infect her with rubella or not. A possible

# A guideline for the new eugenics 83

exception could be when the mother knew she had rubella, and then deliberately became pregnant.

A different exception would be when a lab, hospital or medical profession, for example, has advised a mother that she does not have rubella (or is immune to rubella), after which she then goes ahead and becomes pregnant almost instantly, after which the fetus is affected by rubella after all. There can also be cases in which the mother, for example, uses medication and is told that it is safe, should she become pregnant and then the medication turns out to have some teratogenic action. Such a pregnancy could have been prevented, so the negligence did actually lead to the "damage" in such cases.

Talk about obliging mothers not to smoke, not to use any drugs and not to consume any alcohol during a pregnancy, and criminalizing breaches of such a duty does crop up from time to time. (Gradin v Gradin was a case in Michigan, in which a child sued his mother for having taken drugs during the pregnancy, but the mother was unaware that she was pregnant.) Lawsuits of a child against the mother for negligence during the pregnancy are not allowed in many jurisdictions. In Britain, the Congenital Disabilities Civil Liabilities Act 1976 covers it (makes it impossible), for example.

It is generally thought that the relationship between a mother and her unborn child is so special that to make the mother liable for anything that happens to the fetus would infringe on her rights as an autonomous person. Negligence claims for careless driving with the child in utero have on occasion been upheld, but seem to be covered by motor insurance, in practice. Other than that, these cases are just as controversial as wrongful life claims, as to hold a mother liable would essentially stop women from leading their lives while pregnant.

Here too, the cases center on the need to finance care for the resulting children; see for example the British case CP (A Child) v First-Tier Tribunal (Criminal Injuries Compensation) & Ors.

So far, in wrongful life cases in which courts awarded damages, the essence of the claim is usually wrongful birth, with the difference that the award is made to the child instead of to the parent(s). This can help safeguard the child's care in case the parents die or separate. Questions such as about the parent's right to an informed choice are wrongful birth, not wrongful life considerations.

These cases are often clearly not only linked with the topic of medical malpractice but also with any nation's duty to assist its citizens. That is often the real motivation for wrongful life (and wrongful birth) lawsuits. Perhaps this problem should be addressed through class actions, where possible.

In France, the Perruche case led to new legislation (in 2005) that ensures financial support for families in the event of the disabilities of children, albeit only toward covering basic needs. Britain, for example, was found to be "blatantly discriminatory" against certain groups of disabled or chronically ill citizens by the High Court in December 2017, affecting 1.6 million people but likely benefiting up to 220,000 people in back payments, unfortunately possibly taking several years. The British government had already been informed similarly by a tribunal, but then rewrote the law to avoid having to follow up on that outcome.

This entire discussion also seems to force us to have a discussion about the rights of embryos and fetuses again (see Chapter 7). Does a fetus have a right to life or not? Does a fetus have the same rights as a five-year-old child? Does a fetus have a right not to be harmed? Does a fetus or embryo have the right not to be discriminated against? Can a fetus have a right to be killed?

What does the law say when someone kills a pregnant woman in such a way that the child dies too? Is this one homicide or are these two homicides?

Different jurisdictions deal differently with this question, but a common view appears to be that killing a fetus that is viable outside the womb constitutes fetal homicide. The right to abortion is also often tied to this viability question (and this is about to become muddled, as Glenn Cohen of Harvard has pointed out, with the advent of artificial wombs).

Generally speaking, we do not seem to assign the full set of human rights to fetuses as a prevailing view appears to be that if the mother's life is endangered by the pregnancy, ending the pregnancy is permissible. This is certainly not true in all countries, however. In some countries, such as El Salvador, there are currently problems with the criminalization of women who have had a miscarriage or stillbirth because these women are suspected or accused of having caused the miscarriage or death of the fetus.

## A guideline for the new eugenics

What, however, about children who end up with a life not worth living if this could have been prevented? If I follow my own definitions, such children would have a cause of action in wrongful life cases, as in such cases, life itself could be considered "damage". The "immoral" quality of this conclusion implies that we have a moral duty to apply CRISPR toward the remediation of the related conditions.

Ample support should be provided as a rule, including counseling after the birth of the child if the child turns out to be a non-mainstream child that requires extra support. Ideally, all parents should receive whatever level of support they need. As I've mentioned, I think we'll see a shift in professions in the future that will enable this, for example, considering the immense support males have had in the past, from their spouses, which allowed them to be fully dedicated to their work to a degree that most women still don't have.

Many countries already have support like this in place. If you picture parents having to lift a child all the time and someone needing to be around all the time, you can quickly see that such parents deserve practical and psychological support, not in the least for the child's sake. Such parents require lifting equipment and common sense says that they also need to able to take the occasional evening off and the occasional vacation despite needing to provide the physical care for their child, for instance. In many cases, they would likely require a dedicated carer who is familiar with the child and the circumstances, instead of having to face a new carer every time.

The concept of wrongful life is connected to the idea that this non-discriminatory guideline for the new eugenics obliges us to couple it with euthanasia legislation. Indeed, I believe that we would need to complement such a restrictive (non-discriminatory) eugenics practice as I propose in this book with matching legislation for euthanasia and physician-assisted suicide (see also Appendix D). If we allow someone to come into the world – particularly if that person would have passed away naturally if we hadn't interfered – and that person considers his or her life not worth living as an older child or adult, we must also allow that person to act on that belief. That is only fair. Moreover, I believe that this, too, is part of giving someone the right to live his or her life in dignity.

Keep in mind that even if a person feels that his or her life isn't worth living in the present moment, the hope that this will change in the future, for whatever reason, is usually enough to keep someone from exercising any right to euthanasia or assisted suicide. This is also linked to the moral obligation we have to use techniques like CRISPR first to address conditions that currently still lead to lives "not worth living".

The literature listed at the back of this book contains several examples of actual wrongful life lawsuits, such as the case of Curlender v. Bio-Science Laboratories in the U.S. This concerned a normally conceived child with Tay-Sachs disease, with a life not worth living according to the definition that I propose. The child's parents had undergone blood testing with the specific purpose of assessing whether their offspring was likely to have this condition. Apparently, the lab was somehow negligent in how the blood tests were conducted.

Turpin v. Sortini et al. was a very different case that came before the U.S. courts. The Turpins' first daughter had been examined and tested and incorrectly declared of normal hearing, whereas she was actually completely deaf as the result of a genetic condition. The Turpins then had a second daughter who had the same condition. They stated that had they known about their first child's hereditary deafness, they wouldn't have had the second child.

According to the reasoning I present in this essay, it would have been okay for these parents to decide not to have any further children at all because it cannot be called discriminatory. If the parents tested for the condition in an embryo or fetus and found it present, however, then this should not be a reason to deselect the child as the child would have a life worth living. To decide differently would be discrimination.

To seek damages for emotional distress suffered by these parents (which the Turpins did, among other things), because their child was deaf is also a form of discrimination. A high-IQ child would demand a similar level of care. And who is to say that a hearing child with a normal IQ would require less care? Would the parents have sought damages for emotional distress caused by the fact that they unexpectedly had a child with a high IQ?

In Germany, wrongful life claims are unconstitutional, as such claims would imply that the life of a disabled person is less valuable than that

## A guideline for the new eugenics

of a non-disabled one. The judiciaries in England and Wales, Ontario, and Australia mostly feel the same way.

The Netherlands, on the other hand, has had the case of Kelly Molenaar. This concerned a nine-year-old girl who was born with a serious chromosomal condition, as a result of which she appears to be in constant pain. I think it is fair to see particularly pain as a real impairment as opposed to impairments resulting from hindrances created by society. The child has other problems as well and, for example, has had several heart surgeries. At age two-and-a-half, she had already been admitted to hospital nine times for incessant crying alone, and this was believed to be caused by pain. Kelly's chromosomal condition runs in the family, as a cousin of the father had the same condition and the mother had already had two miscarriages. The medical profession did not follow up on that information, even though the mother had made it available. No family history was taken and there was no consultation with genetics experts. The child's condition was therefore detected too late.

The Court of Appeal in The Hague refused to consider a handicap "damage". However, not only were the parents awarded costs of care and upbringing until the child's 21st birthday, and costs of psychiatric care for the mother after the birth, the court also made the child a party to the case. The case was referred to the Supreme Court (on points of law), which upheld the Court's of Appeal's finding. Kelly was awarded compensation for emotional damage, which would not have occurred if the medical professionals had done their job properly. The court stressed that it had based its damages on the fact that the medical profession had made serious mistakes, not on Kelly's existence as such. After this case, there was a call to ban wrongful life cases in the Netherlands, but no change in the law appears to have come from that. It remains a very difficult topic. In the case of Kelly, one can argue that Kelly's pain could have been prevented and that this is what the Dutch courts mainly based their judgments on. This child is suffering, objectively seen.

France has had the already mentioned successful wrongful life claim of Nicholas Perruche. This concerned a boy born to a mother who contracted rubella during her pregnancy after one of her other children became ill with rubella. In spite of two lab tests and symptoms, the mother was informed that she didn't have rubella and she continued the pregnancy. The French boy's parents brought proceedings on behalf of the boy when he was 6.5 years old. Apparently, he has a heart condition, is deaf as well as blind and may have other neurological conditions. The family first went to court in 1988 and was awarded approximately USD 13,000 (for wrongful birth). The parents, however, also felt that Nicholas himself had been harmed by the laboratory and the physician. Nicholas was awarded damages four times, which was reversed on appeal every time until the case made it to the Cour de Cassation. In this case, too, the medical profession made serious mistakes, but the crux of this case appears to have been financial support for its care and in this case, the award to Nicholas was for the handicaps, in contrast with the Kelly Molenaar case.

France did later (2002) ban wrongful life cases, but it also created a law (2005) that arranges basic care for children like Nicholas Perruche. That is a very important change. Many of these situations hinge on whether or not the parents can look after the child well, in terms of financial means. In the U.S., the parents of Juliana Wetmore not only are looking after their daughter wonderfully well, but they also adopted a child with the same condition (Treacher Collins Syndrome), from another country. Allegedly, it is their Navy-based insurance that makes this possible.

I feel that I do not have enough information to be able to assess whether the cases of Kelly and Nicholas concerned lives not worth living, according to my definition. It certainly appears to be the case for Kelly, but the situation of Nicholas is much less clear and I am not convinced that his life is not worth living.

The cases of Kelly Molenaar and Nicholas Perruche make clear that not only can there be major differences between individual cases, they often have an element of punishment. This is for clear professional negligence (medical malpractice), similar to mistakes like amputating the wrong leg or failing to diagnose cancer that could have been cured if it had been treated instead of misdiagnosed. I think that we have to deal with this separately, not tie it to the lives of the children, however, while nations should step up in the provision of care, the way France has done.

Parents should not be forced to go to court to secure care for their child if that child requires more care (such as multiple surgeries, in the case of Juliana Wetmore) than the average child. Parents should not have to deal with that immense stress. Children (even if only theoretically, considering that the knowledge may remain out of reach of the mental capacity of these children) should never be burdened with the knowledge that their parents felt that they should not have been born.

**We need to talk about this**

## 9. The bioethical imperative

*"We all feel a compelling need to watch stories, to tell stories ... to discuss the things that tell each one of us that we are not alone in the world."*

– Shonda Rhimes

We are not alone in the world. We share the planet with many other species.

Are chickens allowed to live their own lives or should we treat them as inanimate objects even though we know damn well that they're not?

Many people make a distinction about not eating what they call companion animals. Cats, dogs and horses. Those people object to it when Asian people eat dog meat, but don't seem to see a problem with people in the west abusing and eating pigs, cows and chickens. Many people in the western world have chickens as pets. Many keep pigs in the house as pets and some even have pet cows. In some Asian countries, religion does not allow people to eat cows and some religions it is not allowed to eat meat from pigs.

Are people in those countries starting petitions to stop us whities in the west from eating beef, pork, veal and chicken?

This issue is a natural extension from the topics we've talked about in the previous chapters. We are all animals, whether we like it or not. We share the same basic needs with other creatures on the planet. Many of those species have been around much longer than humans. Shouldn't that count for something?

As a geologist, I became highly aware of the striving for equilibrium that drives physical and chemical phenomena (take gravity, for example). As a marine biogeochemist, I developed great awe for the myriad of feedback loops that exist in nature. Once you become aware of that, you start seeing that everything is connected and that almost everything we do as a species has many consequences.

Nature is like this giant multidimensional machine with lots and lots of gearwheels, and when we tweak one of those wheels, it affects many other wheels, usually more wheels than we expect. I am not saying "don't tinker with the wheels". I am saying "be aware that the wheels are connected to many other wheels". I am also saying "Heed the bioethical imperative":

**"All living beings are entitled to respect and should be treated not as a means but as ends in themselves."**

You cannot respect beings without also respecting their habitat, of course. You cannot respect a fish or a dolphin if you poison the water it swims in or keep orcas and dolphins in cruel captivity. You cannot destroy the habitat of other species without needing to remind yourself that this planet is also your own living environment.

I understand the despair of Greta Thunberg very well but at the same time remain a little concerned about the emphasis there still is about climate change. At least, it's increasingly often called that, and not "global warming." We are not only changing climate, but we are also changing the pH of the oceans, we have caused and continue to cause a great deal of chemical pollution, of noise pollution, or light pollution, of pollutions with degradation-resistant artificial materials like plastics that end up in oceans and we have caused a heck of a lot of space pollution.

Whales have trouble hearing themselves over the din we make in waters, birds get lost because our city lights disorient them and other birds are becoming nocturnal so that they can hear each other again. Humans make too much noise during the day.

The arrogance of the human species, and particularly of us whities, knows no bounds.

We consider ourselves superior to all other species.

That, however, is slowly changing. There are habeas corpus cases on behalf of animals and more and more lawyers concern themselves with the rights of other species.

It is also time for us to begin looking at other species differently to see what we can learn from them. In their substantially longer time as species on this planet, they have collected a lot of knowledge that they

## The bioethical imperative

pass on to each other and to their offspring. Some people are quick to scoff at this because non-human animals do not preserve their knowledge in encyclopedias and on hard-disks, but neither did we in the past. That knowledge isn't tangible does not mean that it doesn't exist.

That we speak a different language and are not as good as figuring out the language of animals as (some) animals are at figuring out what human speech means should be more reason for us to give this more thought, not less.

Other species haven't made the messes that the human species has made in such a short time. Who knows what we will discover if we start studying non-human animals from the viewpoint that they may have something to teach. We could find out what their strategies can teach us.

Instead, we continue to pray to the god of speciesism. We are a better species, because. That's why. Because.

I recently read about research with a particular species of bird, in which the researchers had found that these birds helped each other altruistically and these researchers touted this as a major new finding (which it is not, except to the researchers in question). According to the newspaper article, the principal investigator gave as a possible explanation for this kind of behavior that "birds feed their young".

Whether it was the journalist or the researcher who messed up so badly here, it hammers home that we still draw such a strong line between us and other species that it does not even occur to us that the *majority* of species feed their young and that *we do too*. Do we help each other out because we as a species feed our babies? Birds help each other out because it is the right thing to do, also for birds. Because it makes sense.

(I learned a lot about empathy from two parrots and from a pigeon.)

When I was younger, all of us were constantly being told that animals don't play. When we see something that looks like play, scientists said, we were seeing parents teaching their offspring to hunt or we were watching animals catch prey, sometimes very small prey, such as insects, that we simply weren't able to see with our human eyes.

You know that this isn't necessarily entirely true, right?

More and more research is now confirming something that many of us have known for a long time. Animals have emotions. Elephants mourn over the elephant who got killed. Crows may go after the dog or human who attacked one of them weeks or maybe months ago. They also have cognitive abilities. They assess situations and engage in reasoning. They make decisions. They remember things. And if they do all of that, then they're also bound to fool around for no other reason than that they're having fun. Playing.

You know that thing that gulls do, how gulls love to sail on airflows, and sometimes allow a thermal to take them very high up into the sky, circling around and around, and never having to do flap a wing, only making small adjustments?

Well, one day, as I was walking home across the Itchen Bridge in Southampton, I saw a bird hanging in front of that bridge, wings spread, sailing on the upward airflow. Gravity canceled out. The bird was near-stationary. Something was off about it, however, but I was still at some distance so I couldn't put my finger on it.

As I came closer and started climbing the bridge, I saw what was wrong. The bird in question wasn't a gull but a pigeon! I was amazed! I had no idea pigeons did that kind of playful shit too. You could almost hear it yell out loud. "Wheeeeeee!" Just having a good time.

Since then, I have gotten to know pigeons a little better. They're pretty serious birds. They don't have a lot of humor, but they do have abilities that they want to use and if they get very bored they may set themselves goals to reach, challenges to beat the boredom.

They also decide either to commit suicide by car or to retreat to a secluded attic when they feel that their time is up or no longer feel that living is fun. Did you know that? I didn't until only a few years ago.

Did you know that we took them out of their subtropical sea cliff habitats? That we were the ones who spread them all over the world? That they can learn to distinguish between paintings by different painters and music by different composers? That they have many abilities that humans can only dream of? That they recognize our faces while we have the greatest trouble telling them apart unless they have characteristic distinguishing marks?

At the time of writing, British Parliament has just voted to undo

## The bioethical imperative 95

promises made earlier toward child refugees stuck in places like Greece and France, namely to allow them to join relatives who are already in the U.K. The English are great at making promises, pledges and resolutions, but even better at withdrawing them.

We all know what is going to happen to those children. Most of them are going to end up in situations of terrible abuse, sold for sex slavery, child pornography and snuff films. It's Amritsar all over again. This kind of decision has nothing to do with whether or not the human species feeds its own babies. It serves no purpose other than cruelty.

Don't you see the parallel with how we treat other species? Speciesism is a form of otherism. Otherism is when you, for example, firmly believe that cruelty is something only other people engage in. Not you. You could never be cruel. Otherism is when you can justify everything that you do, even refusing vulnerable displaced children the right to join their families and allowing them to become sex slaves and not call it cruelty even though you had promised these children that could come to your country, to their relatives.

Modern society may start to fall apart in as little as thirty years, a recent report said. Is that what the U.K. government is doing without realizing it? Announcing the decline of the human species, in spite of the universal human rights that we drew up together after the Second World War to ensure that what happened during that war would never happen again?

What do you do when you turn a blind eye to child refugees? You effectively give yourself the chance to be able to say later, by way of excuse, *"Wir haben es nicht gewußt."* "We did not know what was going to happen to these children, honestly. We've never had any cases of child abuse in our own country. Child abuse is something only other people engage in, foreign nationals, so we couldn't have known what was going to happen to those children. We could never have imagined that. We're deeply sorry for any alleged harm that may have come to them."

I've also become very aware of the versatility and opportunistic nature of nature.

At the time that this third edition is being published, the world is battling the Covid-19 virus. Is there a message in it, namely to honor the bioethical imperative?

If you consider that poison from plants and animals is either a defense mechanism or an attack mechanism, remember that our over-the-top attempts to kill certain bacteria have made those bacteria resistant and led to superbugs, and realize that many of the new diseases we're seeing have an overlap with habitat destruction or infringement and with the ruthless exploitation of sometimes rare or exotic animals (trading of live animals), you can't escape the thought that diseases like the Covid-19 virus could well serve as a form of biological (natural) defense of non-human animals (with immunity) against humans (with no immunity).

Regardless of whether or not this is true – I don't think it is, not as a purposeful mechanism, but it may be accidentally taking on this role nowadays as a result of what we humans do – please do keep the thought in mind because we can't look at how we treat each other without also scrutinizing how we treat other species. One reflects the other.

# 10. Consequences

*"The roots of education are bitter, but the fruit is sweet."*

– Aristotle

If we want to make the world more inclusive, then there is a lot of room for improvement in several areas, namely medical care and support (and notably financing that care and support), education (of the public at large as well as of experts) and everyday practical matters (housing, offices, shopping, travel and also medicine and policing), which is separate from medical care. The need to couple the non-discriminatory (inclusive) application of the new eugenics with euthanasia legislation should be addressed as well.

To some people, I may sound blissfully unaware of what goes into looking after children and adults who do not fall into the central portions of the population's bell curve. The fact remains that some families are much better able to handle this than others, which could support the idea of turning parenting into a profession or a privilege requiring a license in the distant future. I would not like to see develop the way British Prime Minister Tony Blair envisaged this when he talked about taking children away from parents. The way I see it, babies (embryos) would be created in the lab and assigned randomly; the latter was suggested by Julian Savulescu.

By the time we get to that, many things will have changed in society. We will have made a lot more progress with technologies like CRISPR and there will also be merging of humans with technology that will expand the possibilities of different-bodied people (such as using their brains to operate tools and their living and working environment). If it is true that we will no longer have jobs in the distant future and that all the work and any money that we require will be provided by AI, then we will also have plenty of time to look after each other properly. These are very important development to consider because it means that many reasons that we may see today for applying the new eugenics in a highly discriminatory manner may completely drop away in the future.

At the moment, the need for sufficient time and money to be able to look after one another often translates into us failing to look after each other well. At the moment, making life more inclusive has to include more and better care, not just for the people in the long tail of the human population, but also for the people who look after them (respite care). This will also have to include support for people with temporary or permanent brain-based conditions.

Healthcare and social care is not an area I know a lot about, other than that I can see that these systems seem to be breaking down one after another. Americans generally seem to believe that the British healthcare system is ideal. But not only does your postcode in the U.K. determine whether or not you may get a life-saving medication, but this healthcare system is also breaking down, with some areas even having waiting lists of years just to get seen by a medical specialist.

The Dutch used to have a similar system, the "ziekenfonds", in addition to private insurance for the country's financial elite. They had to abandon it. First, the Dutch introduced fees for medications, which went through years of back-and-forth adjustments. Self-employed people were not in this system, then became incorporated in a way that forced many to switch from that public health care system to private insurance and back all the time, as self-employed people do not have a fixed salary. So, making a business investment one year could push you into the public system the next and back into private insurance with high premiums again the year after that. As far as I know, the Dutch system currently requires that everyone pays monthly premiums, for which the Dutch can get tax credits if their income is low. Many people in the Netherlands now are in arrears, even though they can shop around for their health insurance these days.

I've read that France's healthcare system is good, but such assessments are often made by people who aren't actually using that system and I have no personal experience with it.

Another development is the digitization of healthcare and the introduction of AI. Ilona Kickbush recently pointed out that there is a dark side to the increasing digitalization of health. Among other things, she pointed to Philip Alston's report of October 2019, which he wrote as the UN's Special Rapporteur on extreme poverty and human rights. He observed an increasing drive *"to automate, predict, identify, surveil, detect target and punish"*.

If you are aware of what companies like Facebook, Amazon and Google have been up to, you likely already know that these companies want to track and record you not only via all of your equipment but also through facial recognition wherever you go, and not only want to dictate what you should think and feel, but also want to be your doctor, insurance company, bank and police officer. That's in addition to selling us books, films, groceries, home security and anything else we may want. Will we have to wait and see how this is going to affect our health care? Or is it time to start taking much more responsibility for what happens to us?

Loss of privacy is not necessarily a bad thing, as long as it also holds for the companies who handle our data. The corporate world will have to become fully transparent in how it uses our data. Complete transparency should rule out that our personal data become excuses for raising insurance premiums because that would completely undermine the notion underlying the concept of health insurance.

I think that it will be hard to make any real improvements to how we look after each other without a major shift in our overall approach to life. That would likely be along the lines of what organizations like Extinction Rebellion and PETA are demanding. At first, this may seem out of place here. These issues are all connected, however.

Experts at an Australian think tank have said that if we don't urgently tackle the sorry state our habitat is in and slow down climate change, civilization may start to crumble thirty years from now. If that were to happen, all bets and predictions about health care and support systems will be off and I doubt that we'll ever succeed in making the world more inclusive in that case. We would probably no longer get to have a say about the new eugenics either.

Intuitively, such a doomsday scenario would seem to support my argument that the unbridled use of the new technologies to make our children more competitive from a western capitalist standpoint might lead to the destruction of society. Western capitalism or materialism or consumerism, without any consideration for its effects, including the effects on others, is a major cause of these problems, after all. The collapse of society as a result of climate change would also be the result of that. It would also imply a complete disregard for the one billion people who, according to that Australian report, might be displaced by the effects of climate change.

Make no mistake, however. The problems we are facing are much bigger than climate change alone. We have been forcing ourselves and all wildlife to eat plastic and consume lots of harmful chemicals. We have been displacing, torturing and killing many animals and pushed many into extinction or near-extinction.

All of these areas are connected.

Decades ago, before I went to university, I started reading about Africa and I noticed that we arrogant whities went there, telling the people living there what to do and to stop doing what they were doing as if they didn't know their own lands best and we whities seem to have set a string of problems in motion there. Fairly recently, I saw research in which Dutch scientists expressed surprise that the African farmers in their project did not select the biggest plots of land but wanted the best ones. We also have a giant modern slavery problem; modern slavery is estimated to be the fate of 40 million people around the world. As long as we keep doing this kind of thing to each other, keep seeing some people as lesser humans, we will keep shooting ourselves in the foot as a species because you can't look after the human habitat well without caring about every creature in it.

A second area that needs a boost is education about diversity, not just education of members of the public but also of bioethics experts, medical professionals, architects, landscape and city planners, shop and furniture designers, police officers and others to help eradicate stigmas and to enable people to live their lives with fewer practical hindrances.

A major push for change in that area has to come from the healthcare professions, as they are currently still among the main propagators of health-related stigmas, along with police officers and judges. When health professionals, for example, write "refused follow-up consultations" in their patient file instead of "declined" and do not include the information that the person in question will be 200 miles away at the time of those proposed follow-ups, they are keeping mental health stigma alive by depicting a mental health patient as obstinate and refusing to cooperate.

When supermarkets still stock magazines of which the cover prominently features the suggestion that parents of autistic children might want to "fire up" their children's brains, you know that whoever wrote that headline hasn't got a clue as to what autism is.

Schools should have the topic of diversity in the curriculum. Children should get to discover how many different ways there are to communicate with others. Businesses should become familiar with the benefits of employing people who are a little bit different just like they also had to get used to the idea of employing women instead of only men. Just like all homes to be built from now on should have the lowest possible energy requirement and provide the highest possible wellbeing such as by using "passive house" techniques, all buildings should also be as inclusive as possible from the start so that they won't need to be especially adapted. Combating domestic violence and war is also recommended. These are things that we can simply decide to do. All it requires is our will and determination.

At the moment, notably different-bodied people but also different-brained people experience lots of practical hindrances when they want to shop or use public transport. People who make a train journey in a wheelchair can't always rely on being able to get onto or off a train. They are sometimes even told to stay on the train and take another train back because that second train will be better equipped for letting them descend onto the station platform.

The education we need also demands good communication between the specialists and the public. It's definitely not the case that only the public needs to be educated. Scientists and other specialists have their biased, flaws and blind spots too. There are, for example, quite a few science writers, philosophers and bioethicists who feel that the public is often intimidated by technological progress or distrusts it. They may say that such people have an innate trust in everything "natural" and that they feel only the natural is good. I think that the opposite also applies. People who believe that the public is intimidated by science and technology may feel threatened by the natural variation among humans and fail to see that this rich diversity constitutes genuine wealth. The debate is not even about nature on one side against science and technology on the other side.

In his 2001 article "Procreative beneficence: Why we should select the best children", Julian Savulescu mentioned "desires" that according to him are "based on irrational fears (e.g., about interfering with nature or playing God)" as one reason why "couples do not want to use or obtain available information about genes which will affect well-being". He essentially argued that we should see children like products, prizes or rewards because he compared them to boxes on Wheel of Fortune. Although that article is now almost two decades old, Savulescu did not appear to have changed his views greatly as he has said similar things in various interviews and publications since then.

In a 2015 interview with journalist and philosopher Bas Heijne for Dutch VPRO TV, he said of Michael Sandel, Jürgen Habermas, Leon Kass and Francis Fukuyama that they are against enhancing normal human beings (as opposed to curing diseases), and called this with a snarky chuckle, a "really a pre-scientific view of nature and the evolution of human beings". I don't get why he so often seems to feel that it is necessary to add sneers and chuckles with regard to anyone who does not hold the exact same views as he does.

Similarly puzzling is his obsession with "psychopaths", a word that he uses in almost every other sentence without specifying it, and his paranoia about the backyard laboratories in which according to him, 1% of the human population might be creating biological weapons of mass destruction. Psychopathic traits are common among internet trolls and some hackers, but to my (limited) knowledge, Savulescu has never mentioned trolls or hackers, or neuroscientist James Fallon.

Is this the point at which I should accuse Savulescu of a cognitive bias?

The problem with Savulescu's brash style and nonsensical statements is that they can obscure the little gems that he sometimes produces as well. He has suggested the handing out of embryos randomly to people, which is in line with Sandel's way of thinking. This is not only brilliant, it's already proven to be a viable concept as people have already adopted random other people's embryos to create so-called snow babies. Together with Peter Singer, Savulescu wrote an article in which he and Singer commented on the He Jiankui case. It was surprising to see that in essence, they appear to agree with the spirit of the guideline that I have proposed in this book.

A great deal of improvement is also needed in the practical realm (besides care and how we finance it). People who make a train journey in a wheelchair can't always rely on being able to get onto or off a train. They are sometimes even told to stay on the train and take another train back that is better equipped for letting them descend onto the station platform.

We need a change in the medical community, and this is linked to educating medical professionals about diversity. The limitations we have had with regard to accepting diversity also mean that traditional medicine is flawed by definition unless you're a white mainstream male. Clinical trials used to contain only white mainstream males. Even women were excluded, notably menstruating women because including them would complicate the picture too much (gendered medicine). So we now have the reality that the medications doctors prescribe may often work well for white mainstream males, but not so much if you're a woman, part of an ethnic minority or aren't neurotypical.

Traditional medicine is also eugenic. It sees a standardized body and standardized behaviors as something to strive for. We also see this reflected in preferences for hearing aids over learning sign language and risky spine surgeries over more advanced wheelchairs. There is even a wheelchair for deep-sea diving. Normal-bodied people see wheelchairs as limitations, but the people who use them often have an opposite view of them. Do you remember when you got your first car or got your driving license? Isn't driving a car also a limitation relative to a jaguar, who doesn't need a car to be able to go fast or a pigeon or pelican, who does not need a jet plane? It has not stopped us from using cars.

We need to come up with a system in which all humans can get all the care they need and want. We need to build a world in which everyone is allowed and enabled to flourish to the best of her or his abilities and wishes.

**We need** to talk about this

# 11. Lessons from the past and present

*"Some of the best lessons we ever learn are learned from past mistakes. The error of the past is the wisdom and success of the future."*

– Dale Turner

### APPENDIX A: EXAMPLES OF OLD-STYLE EUGENICS

#### Austria

As recently as 1997, Austria still sterilized mentally handicapped women, most often against their will.

#### Australia

At the end of 2015, The Guardian published an article reporting that the UN were examining Australia's practice of forced sterilization of women with disabilities. The article included the example of a 39-year-old woman who was sterilized at age seven because she had a vision impairment.

Forced sterilization of Aboriginal women and children may still occur today as well. In the past, Australia treated aboriginals like wild animals or cattle. It also removed large numbers of Aboriginal children from their families and, for example, placed them in dormitories. Aboriginal people with disabilities made and likely still make up a large proportion of Australia's prison population.

#### Belgium

Still fairly recently, Belgium sterilized women who were deemed physically or mentally inferior (although it never had a systematic sterilization program). One of these women was Ingrid Van Butsel. She was not allowed to marry her husband in 1985 unless she submitted to sterilization. Supposedly, she was threatened with being hospitalized in a psychiatric institution if she didn't give in. Although not disabled, she was raised among mentally and physically disabled children after her mother succumbed to tuberculosis. Her intelligence is slightly above average for Flemish women in her age group.

In 1997, a Belgian bioethics committee advised the government minister for health that standard forced sterilization of mentally handicapped persons should never be allowed, and that a multidisciplinary team of people should advise any physician wanting to carry out the sterilization of a mentally handicapped person in incidental cases.

**Britain**

Modern ideas of eugenics first popped up in 19th-century Britain, proposed by Francis Galton. From there, they appear to have spread to the United States, particularly but not exclusively California, which in turn inspired Adolf Hitler in Germany.

Forced sterilization of women with for example learning disabilities currently occasionally takes place in Britain. In the practice of assisted reproductive technologies (ART) in Britain, it is also essentially forbidden by law to implant pre-embryos that test positive for certain conditions.

Although the following are not examples of eugenics, they are examples of social engineering, which is related.

1. Fetuses are sometimes removed through C-sections (cesarean), occasionally even from foreign women who are merely passing through a British airport or are visiting Britain, as happened to Alessandra Pacchieri, an Italian woman with bipolar disorder, in 2012. Her baby was adopted by a British couple a year later. Note that strong hormone fluctuations also can temporarily impair women who do not have bipolar disorder but for example a myoma. Why should bipolar women be treated differently when hormone fluctuations temporarily affect them? Occurrences such as these (including a large number of forced adoptions of children taken away from couples living in Britain) tend to take place in complete secrecy, and often include gag orders for the parents. These cases are now increasingly brought into the open, however, as a result of pressure from the press and other parties, but also particularly under the encouragement of Britain's highest family law judge, Sir James

## Lessons from the past and present 107

Munby (who recently retired).

2. Prime Minister Tony Blair argued in a BBC interview in 2006 that the decision should be made to take children away from certain parents, even before birth, for example, if he felt that those children would only grow up to become "hooligans" later. Blair even set and then increased national "adoption targets" for municipalities between 2000 and 2006.

3. Social cleansing also takes place in London, where families are removed and rehoused at great distances and where some buildings have two types of entrances, one for wealthy tenants and one for poor tenants, the latter at the back. (Allowing a few poor tenants to live in a building as well can have financial advantages for developers because it can help them get planning permission, though this may change after Brexit.)

On 11 January 2018, The Guardian reported that a secret eugenics meeting had been taking place at University College London at which allegedly white supremacists were present. Apparently, it hadn't been the first of those meetings either. As I was wrapping up the previous edition of this book, I noticed a storm of protest on Twitter regarding what a self-proclaimed Tory character called Toby Young apparently had said on BBC Radio 4 about "progressive eugenics".

Various Tory politicians have also made remarks suggesting that sterilizing poor people should be mandatory. In February 2020, as I was wrapping up the present edition, Andrew Sabisky, a newly appointed advisor to the British Prime Minister (Boris Johnson) resigned. Not only had he turned out to be racist and sexist, he too entertained old-style eugenics ideas. Some of the Tories who come up with these ideas don't realize what poverty is, what causes it and what it results in. Remarks such as that poor people should not go to a food bank, but take out a payday loan at exorbitant interest rates (for which they might not even qualify) drive home that the Tories who make these remarks are either "taking the mickey" (making fun of the poor) or completely, eh, delusional. Their class thinking hampers them greatly. Poverty is not the result of low intelligence, but is usually the result of government actions.

(For those in other countries, British food banks used to provide up to three packages of emergency food for about three days, per year. That was raised to a maximum of six packages per year, so they don't compare to food banks in, for example, the Netherlands, where food banks aim to uphold a certain standard of living as opposed to merely helping people stay alive. British food banks are vital and have brought many Brits to tears out of sheer gratitude. Unlike what many people assume, the threshold to a food bank is huge. If you have children to feed, you have no choice, but most people avoid going to a food bank as long as possible.)

## Canada

It is now known that indigenous women (who often have large families, just like my Dutch grandparents) were being pressured into sterilization in Saskatoon. Among them was Brenda Pelletier, who underwent the procedure in 2010. Melika Popp was sterilized in 2008. Pressure was also put on Tracy Bannab in 2012. The Saskatoon Health Region apologized and changed its policies.

In 1928, the "Sexual Sterilization Act" came into force in Alberta and it wasn't repealed until 1972. It permitted the sterilization of persons discharged from mental institutions because criminality, mental illness, and immorality were seen as strongly heritable and objectionable. It resulted in the sterilization of 2,832 persons.

## Germany

Approximately 11 million people were killed during World War II because they were deemed undesirable within the framework of creating a human super race. This widespread extreme practice of eugenics did not only victimize Jews, but also Poles, Roma gypsies and other Slavs (notably Ukrainians and Byelorussians), persons with physical or mental disabilities, Jehovah's Witnesses, alcoholics, homosexuals, dissenting clergy, prostitutes, communists, socialists and other people with dissenting political views.

In 1934, 300,000 to 400,000 people were forcibly sterilized, mainly those in mental health hospitals and other institutions. The Nazis began killing people with physical and mental handicaps in 1939.

Most people associate the word "eugenics" with these Nazi practices and with the ideas of Nazi leader Adolf Hitler. Among other things, the Nazis introduced the Law for the Prevention of Hereditarily Diseased Offspring in 1933.

### India

India currently appears to have the practice of forcing women into camps where they are sterilized. The matter recently gained international attention when 60 women fell ill and at least 12 died after a mass sterilization event.

### Japan

About 25,000 people were sterilized without consent between 1948 and 1996. Japan currently also requires transgender candidates to be sterilized before they can transition. Japan is facing pressure from the United Nations, the World Health Organization and others to abolish this demand.

### Peru

In 1996, then-president Alberto Fujimori launched a sterilization program. Although it began with positive intentions and was initially received well, more and more women eventually appear to have been sterilized without their consent. Most of them were poor and indigenous.

### Scandinavia

Denmark, Finland, Norway and Sweden introduced eugenics laws in the 1930s.

In Sweden, 60,000 young women deemed mentally defective or otherwise "incapable of looking after their children" were pressured or forced into sterilization between 1936 and 1976. The reasoning behind it seems to have been threefold:

1. So-called feeble-minded and insane people were supposed to breed more freely than thrifty and energetic people of "superior" stock.

2. The government wanted to be "kind" to people who needed

"protection" against propagating their own "weak" genes.

3. The government wanted to save the state the heavy cost of welfare for "the very dim".

The Danish sterilized 11,000 people for similar reasons between 1929 and 1967. The Norwegians and Finns each forcibly sterilized around 1,000 women in roughly the same period.

Finland requires transgenders first to be diagnosed with a mental disorder and then to be sterilized if a person wants his or her (trans)gender legally recognized.

**United States**

Federally funded sterilization programs took place in 32 states throughout the 20th century. Their goal was to control the populations of "undesirables" such as immigrants, people of color, poor people, unmarried mothers, and the physically and mentally disabled.

California led these developments, with more than 20,000 Californian men and women in institutions being sterilized between roughly 1909 and 1979, often without their full knowledge and consent. (Apparently, Adolf Hitler – see "Germany" – got his inspiration from California.) The main idea was to eliminate characteristics thought to be associated with "conditions" such as criminality, feeble-mindedness and sexual deviance. Asians and Mexicans were also particularly targeted.

Southern states targeted sterilization at African Americans. North Carolina also targeted women seen as "delinquent" or "unwholesome". In the 1930s, Virginia targeted people deemed feeble-minded and unfit to reproduce, such as the so-called Brush Mountain people.

Forced sterilization of Native Americans took place as well. It was estimated that as many as 25 to 50 percent of Native American women were sterilized just between 1970 and 1976 alone.

Puerto Rico experienced forced sterilizations on a major scale.

Many states in the U.S. currently also require transgenders to be sterilized.

# Lessons from the past and present

### Switzerland

Switzerland forcibly sterilized mentally handicapped people on the basis of a 1928 sterilization law. This was challenged in 1997 by the National Council of the Women of Switzerland, which called for a government investigation.

Since I compiled this list, many more cases of unacceptable eugenic practices that are still taking place in the present or that were applied fairly recently have come to light.

**We need to talk about this** 112

## APPENDIX B: EXAMPLES OF WHEN PROGRESS BACKFIRED

### Thalidomide

Thalidomide was a sedative prescribed to suppress the nausea that tends to accompany pregnancy. It was believed safe. It caused limb deformations as well as malformations of the cardiovascular, intestinal and urinary systems of the affected babies and was taken off the market in the early 1960s. (I could have been a thalidomide baby.) Thalidomide was marketed under various trade names. In humans, a small dose is enough to have these teratogenic effects, whereas it takes much larger quantities before it causes damage to the offspring of other species. Fortunately, it was later able to gain a new reputation, as notably an anticancer drug, but in its original role, it affected over 10,000 fetuses. Those who've been around long enough may remember photos of the resulting babies in newspaper articles.

### DDT and other pesticides

DDT (1,1,1-trichloro-2,2-bis(4-chlorophenyl)ethane, or dichlorodiphenyltrichloroethane), aldrin, dieldrin, and lindane are examples of pesticides that were introduced and later banned. DDT causes nerve damage and affects the hormone-producing systems of many animals, among other things lowering their fertility. DDT was initially lauded as a miracle pesticide and insecticide, and a Nobel Prize was awarded in connection with it, but there had been concerns about it from the beginning. It was the environmentalist and marine biologist Rachel Carson's work that eventually led to a ban on DDT and other pesticides in the United States. Among other things, DDT almost eradicated the bald eagle in the United States after it had already been hunted and killed relentlessly on the grounds of myths about the damage the bird did to agriculture.

Today, DDT is still used to control the spreading of malaria in some areas. At the time of writing of this book, groups of people all over the world are fighting to get other harmful pesticides banned, such as glyphosate and chlorpyrifos. That isn't because they're afraid of progress. It's because they use their brains and aren't narrow-sighted. They are following in Rachel Carson's footsteps, and we know now that she was right.

In 1984, methyl isocyanate from a pesticide plant in Bhopal, India accidentally killed more than 3500 people and exposed more than 500,000 to the toxic gas.

### PCBs

Polychlorinated biphenyls (PCBs) are very stable compounds that were used as plasticizers, coolants, and in many other ways. These toxic compounds accumulate particularly in the fatty tissues of animals, affecting for example seabirds. Countries began banning them in the 1970s.

### CFCs

CFCs (chlorofluorocarbons) and the bromine-based halons were used as solvents and coolants, as well as in the production of various (packaging) foams, among other things. They seemed harmless until we discovered that they were destroying the stratospheric ozone layer that protects us against getting too much UV from the sun and limits the incidence of skin cancer.

### Dioxins

Agent Orange and Seveso are perhaps the best-known names in connection with dioxins. The dioxins consist of two groups of chemicals, the PCDDs and the PCDFs (polychlorinated dioxins and polychlorinated dibenzofurans). Dioxins form when for instance PVC burns incompletely in a waste incinerator, but this is not the only way by which dioxins can end up in the environment. Dioxins are also connected with herbicides, for example. The formulation Agent Orange was used in warfare to cause trees and shrubs to lose their leaves and contained dioxin proper (TCDD). It affected many people who handled it. TCDD was also released in massive quantities during an industrial incident in the Italian town of Seveso in 1976. Dioxins have multiple negative effects on human health, such as on the immune system, the endocrine system and reproductive functions. At least one dioxin is classified as a known human carcinogen.

### DES

DES babies may be a term many people my age may be familiar with as it potentially affected us. DES (diethylstilbestrol) was given to pregnant women to prevent early labor and miscarriages. It did not prevent such complications, but did cause tumors and other effects, none of which were desirable, particularly for children exposed to DES in the uterus.

### Antibiotics

The effects of the overuse of antibiotics (another version of "life killers") are well known. As microorganisms increasingly develop resistance to antibiotics (also because they end up in sewage plants via our toilets), antibiotics now make it increasingly harder to treat infections in people who desperately need them. That's because we have been prescribing them in great numbers to people who don't need them and feeding them to commercially exploited livestock as a prophylactic measure, thereby encouraging the development of resistant strains.

### Chloroform, bromoform and other compounds

Chloroform and bromoform were habitually used as, for example, solvents until their toxicity became clear. They are carcinogenic and toxic to the liver. The octane booster MTBE, which replaced methylene chloride, had problems too. Many of the compounds used in the chemical cleaning sector suffered from similar toxicity difficulties.

### Flame retardants

Brominated flame retardants ended up everywhere in the environment, even in the tissues of polar bears in the Arctic, and also had to be phased out.

### PFAS

Both the household use and production of fluorine-based non-stick coatings (PTFE, polytetrafluoroethylene, Teflon) for kitchenware and as heat-resistant coatings in for example space heaters, heat lamps and hairdryers are problematic as well. While PTFE certainly has its usefulness, for example in laboratories (I've used Teflon labware) and hospital settings, and also as a lubricant, both its manufacture and its household use raise questions.

Accidental overheating of non-stick cookware can result in the release of several extremely toxic compounds. It has led to the agonizing deaths of many pet birds, and PTFE overheating has also killed large numbers of poultry. The respiratory systems of birds are much more sensitive than those of mammals, but the compounds released during first heating or overheating of PTFE affect human health as well. Problem chemicals are also involved in the manufacture of PTFE.

Perfluorooctanoic acid (PFAO), also known as C8, dissolves well in water and does not decay in any way. It is now globally present in the air and in seawater. In the Netherlands, discharges by the Chemours plant in Dordrecht led to increased PFOA concentrations in the Merwede river and in the groundwater along its banks. In the U.S., a former DuPont plant in West Virginia released more than 1.7 million pounds of C8 into the region's water, soil and air between 1951 and 2003.

C8 was phased out after a class-action lawsuit that alleged that it causes cancer. Chemours now makes a new compound called GenX instead, for which safety thresholds have yet to be established. Regular water treatment methods don't remove it from drinking water. GenX may be safer than C8, but it is also alleged to have caused tumors and reproductive problems in lab animals. In some locations, GenX has already freely been released into the environment for decades as a result of a flaw in the legislation.

Here are two questions that I would like to see answered:

1. What have non-stick coatings on cookware brought us? I haven't used non-stick pots and pans in years and that works just fine. Heat lamps and space heaters seem to function fine without these coatings too. (And why are there no automatic temperature switches on stovetops? Overheating of for example an electric stovetop accidentally left on has caused plenty of small fires.)

2. Why is there no sticker on products that indicates whether or

## Lessons from the past and present

not they contain PTFE? I have a toaster that may contain the stuff. If I use something that harbors a potential health risk, whether for me, my pets or my family members, shouldn't I know about it? Shouldn't I have a choice as to whether or not I buy or use PTFE?

Have you heard of "forever chemicals"? That's what this is about. These forever chemicals caused a bit of a crisis in the Netherlands in 2019, when new legal guidelines for maximum allowable contents of PFAS in notably soil brought many construction projects to a halt because the stuff is everywhere. There are approximately 6,000 PFAS compounds (perfluoroalkyl and polyfluoroalkyl substances).

The answers lie in commercial interests. In practice, they often weigh heavier than our health. The manufacturers of these coatings – initially intended for use in space flight – have known for a long time that there are risks associated with the manufacturing as well as with the use.

(IVF is also a big commercial market that continues to grow rapidly. Pharmaceutics is big business. Whose interests will be at the foreground of new developments in human procreation?)

### Smoking

You may also ponder the fact that in 1960, 58% of American men and 36% of American women were smokers. In those days, smoking four packets of cigarettes per day was considered fine (but Big Tobacco knew better). Four years later, we slowly started reversing that notion and tobacco products now all carry health warnings. Smoking remained cool for a long time in spite of the clear health risks and in the late 1970s, you were still often considered a klutz if you didn't smoke.

### Plastics

Plastic is taking up more and more space in the oceans and we'll soon have more plastic than fish in the oceans. We have microplastics in our blood. Honey has microplastics in it too, and microplastics have also been found in bottled water, drinking water and beer. Where does a large portion of those microplastics come from? Our clothes and carpets.

Another major part is derived from larger objects. Look at the albatrosses whose bellies are filled with plastic bottle caps, at remote locations. Look at all the shorelines littered with so many kinds of plastic. Yes, we are now starting to develop sugar-based biodegradable plastic bottles that are much stronger than plastic bottles and new biobased fibers, but isn't it a little late for that? Why did we never ask what would happen with our plastic waste after we discarded our disposable and durable plastic products? Did we really never consider that?

Never?

Clearly, we humans are neither omniscient nor clairvoyant.

## Nanoparticles

We are now using nanoparticles on a significant scale – your toothpaste may contain them – yet we don't have any technologies that can separate them from waste streams. Have you ever asked yourself what these tiny particles do to our organs? Speaking of toothpaste, I now use baking soda instead, and I choose a brand that comes packaged in paper and cardboard. It's considerably cheaper than toothpaste, brings down my plastic waste output a tiny little bit, and also seems to make my teeth much less sensitive to low temperatures. For dental cleaning, it works just as well, also according to dentists.

One of my colleagues probably won't thank me for saying this, but I am more worried about nanoparticles than about the new eugenics. I suspect that nanoparticles have the potential to wipe us out because I see them as potentially affecting biology like sand thrown into an engine or machinery. Biology may be able to cope with them fine, but I wonder at what cost to each organism. We also don't know how they may affect microorganisms, many of which we depend on (those in our gut, for instance, but also in various stages of food production). We have very little if any control over nanoparticles and they get into everything, including our organs. They offer great possibilities in medicine, however. Thankfully, I am not up to date on nanoparticles, so I keep telling myself that my knowledge is probably simply hopelessly outdated.

# Lessons from the past and present

## Dams

We also used to see dams as useful by definition. They created water reservoirs and we sometimes used the water to drive turbines in power plants. But top water management experts no longer consider dams particularly good because dams block sediment flow. China, Germany and the Netherlands are examples of countries that are experiencing challenges because of dams. Today's approach to river management is a much more natural one ("building with nature"). Ask the Dutch, whose lowland delta country with rivers like the Rhine and Meuse discharging into a sea has made them intimately familiar with marine and fluvial flooding, which has put them at the forefront of water management insights. And what about the villagers who were forced out of their homes to make way for dammed reservoirs and the wildlife displaced destroyed in the process?

## Electronic technology

In The Guardian on 8 February 2018, David Smith reported about a plea made at a conference in Washington to companies like Facebook. "The leaders of Facebook," it said, "should consider children when they make decisions that could harm millions of young people hooked on the social network." Silicon Valley alumni, former tech workers turned whistleblowers, including people like Roger McNamee (an early investor in Facebook, now part of the Center for Humane Technology), and lobbyists are issuing warnings about "potential links between tech addiction and sleep disruption, poor academic performance, anxiety, depression, obesity, social isolation and suicide". James Steyer of Common Sense Media organized the meeting. He promotes safe technology and media for children while criticizing companies like Google, Twitter and Facebook. In Davos in January 2018, Marc Benioff of Salesforce, "called for Facebook to be regulated like a cigarette company because of the addictive and harmful properties of social media."

## Water, food, space litter, sugar, breast implants

Why do we still use drinking water to flush our toilets? Why are we only now willing to concede that myopia (near-sightedness) may have something to do with forcing kids to focus predominantly on short distances (writing, reading, and now typing and staring at mobile gadgets), an idea dismissed as utterly ridiculous not that long ago? Why do the households in any western country buy excessive quantities of food that they throw out one or two weeks later to the tune of billions of pounds, euros or dollars per year? And did you see that recent image showing the gigantic amount of space litter that now circles the planet? It's crazy!

Need I go on? Need I mention the various types of dangerous breast implants we've had, for example? Toxic dental fillings? The neurotoxin monosodium glutamate (E621)? (Oh, that lovely feeling as if you've been run over by a big truck the day before.) Sugar, and some kids already needing liver transplants as a result of too much sugar in their diets? The cases of industrial aluminum, chromium and other kinds of metal poisoning and the Erin Brokoviches of the world who expose them? There are many more examples of how we got things wrong in the past.

My point is that we humans clearly really aren't as smart as we think we are (and we are not very good at predicting what we don't know yet). Maybe the strongest indicator of that is that we humans haven't actually been on the planet very long yet but have already done more damage to our own habitat than any other species. Birds, for example, have roamed the planet much longer than we have. But birds don't care about money. Humans appear to have a strong tendency to let money dictate what happens. Commercial interests steamroller all over us until damage – harm – becomes clear and the voices of protest grow louder. I wish that weren't true. I like progress. I like technological advancements. I like cool new stuff. It's exciting what we can do. Until we start looking at the other side of progress. Apparently, we have about two decades in which we can still turn the overall decline of our habitat around in terms of biodiversity. Two decades. Twenty years. That's the time that passed between my birth and my first real job, in Amsterdam.

I am not afraid of progress and I am not afraid of chemicals either. I have not only handled Teflon labware, but also bromoform, boiling hot concentrated acids, radioactive materials and even osmium tetroxide in the lab and none of that has given me sleepless nights. But we shouldn't be producing massive numbers of toxins, and releasing them into the environment, expecting them to have no ill effects on our lives whatsoever. And so on and so forth.

## APPENDIX C: TRENDS OF EMANCIPATION

Here are some dates and data that may inspire.

1689:

Female landowners are allowed to vote in elections to the States of Friesland in rural districts. Friesland is now part of the Netherlands, has its own language.

1799:

John Chavis is the first black person on record to attend an American college or university, at what is now Washington and Lee University in Lexington, Virginia. There is no record of a degree.

1823:

Alexander Lucius Twilight becomes the first known African American to graduate from a college in the United States. He received a bachelor's degree from Middlebury College in Vermont.

1841:

Abraham Lincoln, who is still a young lawyer at that point, wins a Supreme Court case in Illinois, which frees Nance Legins-Costley from "indentured servitude", thereby also setting her son free, presumed to be the first black male slave who was freed.

1863:

Abraham Lincoln, as president of the U.S., issues the Emancipation Proclamation, which declares all slaves in rebel states that are not under Union control to be free.

1870:

The first woman is admitted to Cornell University in the U.S.

1871:

Harriette Cooke becomes the first female college professor in the U.S., a full professor with a salary equal to that of the male professors.

1893:

New Zealand is the first self-governing colony in the world in which all women are given the right to vote in parliamentary elections. However, women barred from standing for election until 1919.

1920:

Oxford starts awarding degrees to women. Women had studied and completed degrees at Oxford since the 1870s. Men had had full access for centuries. (Italy, on the other hand, was very early with giving women access to universities and degrees.)

1933:

Franklin Roosevelt becomes America's first president who uses a wheelchair. His disability is mostly kept hidden from the public. He is elected to more terms than any other U.S. president.

1964:

Women are allowed to vote in Libya, Papua New Guinea (Territory of Papua and Territory of New Guinea), and Sudan.

1966:

Women are allowed to vote in the Swiss canton of Basel-Stadt.

## Lessons from the past and present 123

1971:

Women can vote in Switzerland (federal level).

1980:

Women can vote in Iraq.

1980:

Guion Bluford becomes the first black astronaut to go into space in 1983. At least, that's what they say. But it had actually happened three years earlier, on a Russian Soyuz spacecraft, and it was Arnaldo Tamayo Méndez, a Cuban of African descent.

1984:

Women can vote in Liechtenstein.

1991:

The Federal Supreme Court of Switzerland forces the Swiss canton of Appenzell Innerrhoden to accept women's suffrage. Women can now vote.

2006:

Katie Apostolides, a woman born with Down syndrome, studies art with a major in education at Becker College, a small liberal arts school in Massachusetts.

2007:

Brittney Exline enrolls as a freshman student at the University of Pennsylvania, at age 15. This makes her the youngest African-American female ever to enroll at an Ivy League university.

2009:

Barack Obama becomes the first non-white and the first black U.S. president.


2012:

Otis Kryzanauskas, Canada's first male midwife, graduates with a bachelor of sciences in midwifery from McMaster University.


2012:

Ido Kedar, an autistic guy who spent the first half of his life completely trapped in silence, publishes his first book, Ido in Autismland.

He had to fight to get an education, but succeeded, graduated high school with a diploma and a 3.9 GPA. He is continuing his education in college.

He communicates by typing on an iPad or a letter board. He later publishes a second book, In Two Worlds, which is a novel.


2013:

A Kentucky woman with Down syndrome graduates from a technical college.


2013:

Ángela Bachiller, a woman born with Down syndrome, is sworn in as city councilor for the Spanish city of Valladolid.


2014:

Ezra Roy, a man born with Down syndrome, graduates magna cum laude from Texas Southern University, with a bachelor's degree with art as his major and a minor in theatre.

## Lessons from the past and present

2015:

Women's suffrage is introduced in Saudi Arabia along with the right to run for municipal elections.

2016:

Hope Banks, a woman born with Down syndrome, graduates from college in the U.S.

2017:

AnneCatherine Heigl, a cheerleader from Zionsville, Indiana who was born with Down syndrome, is accepted to George Mason University.

2018:

Odette Harris becomes the first black woman professor of neurosurgery in the U.S., at Stanford.

2018:

Jonny Peay, a man born with Down syndrome, is accepted to Utah State University.

2018:

Nicolas Joncour directs a video, which is published online. He is a pianist, a nonspeaking autistic and a university student in France. He types to communicate. He earlier wrote an article about his right to an education.

2018:

A café in Japan starts experimenting with using robots remotely operated by people with severe physical disabilities.

Not that long ago, we thought that people like Nico and Ido were not capable of anything much and stuck them in asylums where we deprived them of development, interactions, opportunities, life's normal experiences and isolated them, treated them badly, and worse. (Actually, we still do, also in Britain.) We used to do the same thing to people who were born with Down syndrome and still often do it and to many others, such as people who are gay.

We did something similar to women and to all people who had different skin tones other than "white".

Now we are even starting to acknowledge that we can't do this to chimpanzees, elephants, cattle, geese, pigs, ducks and chickens either, and the legal rights of animals and even rivers, mountains and lakes are being developed. We still have a long way to go, but when we look back, we can see that we've made progress too

## APPENDIX D: GRONINGEN PROTOCOL

### The Groningen Protocol for euthanasia in newborns

**Requirements that must be fulfilled**

- The diagnosis and prognosis must be certain
- Hopeless and unbearable suffering must be present
- The diagnosis, prognosis, and unbearable suffering must be confirmed by at least one independent doctor
- Both parents must give informed consent
- The procedure must be performed in accordance with the accepted medical standard

**Information needed to support and clarify the decision about euthanasia**

*Diagnosis and prognosis*

- Describe all relevant medical data and the results of diagnostic investigations used to establish the diagnosis
- List all the participants in the decision-making process, all opinions expressed, and the final consensus
- Describe how the prognosis regarding long-term health was assessed
- Describe how the degree of suffering and life expectancy were assessed
- Describe the availability of alternative treatments, alternative means of alleviating suffering, or both
- Describe treatments and the results of treatment preceding the decision about euthanasia

*Euthanasia decision*

- Describe who initiated the discussion about possible euthanasia and at what moment
- List the considerations that prompted the decision
- List all the participants in the decision-making process, all opinions expressed, and the final consensus
- Describe the way in which the parents were informed and their opinions

*Consultation*

- Describe the physician or physicians who gave a second opinion (name and qualifications)
- List the results of the examinations and the recommendations made by the consulting physician or physicians

*Implementation*

- Describe the actual euthanasia procedure (time, place, participants, and administration of drugs)
- Describe the reasons for the chosen method of euthanasia

*Steps taken after death*

- Describe the findings of the coroner
- Describe how the euthanasia was reported to the prosecuting authority
- Describe how the parents are being supported and counseled
- Describe planned follow-up, including case review, postmortem examination, and genetic counseling

## 12. Afterword

*"Gems exist by the grace of light. If you don't see any gems, something may be blocking the light."*

– Angelina Souren

After the previous versions of this book, it occurred to me that I should paint a picture of a possible future. After the world ground to a halt after He Jiankui's announcement, I can now funnily enough actually envision a scenario such as described in my guideline happening in real life.

In Chapters 7 and 8, I have explained how I arrived at this horribly "calculative" guideline that focuses on the individuals receiving CRISPR and other treatments. It has little to do with personal preferences.

In fact, if I allowed myself to be motivated by personal experiences, I would probably want to focus on lung cancer because lung cancer is often a horrible way to go, and is often detected too late. But then, heart disease and colon disease or muscular diseases or Alzheimer's can also impact people's lives badly. None of those have happened in my family, as far as I know, but there've been three cases of lung cancer. Progressive MS is another disease that I would love to see tackled. But if I had allowed myself to be motivated personally, it would have been hard to find a logical, stepwise progression that we might follow as a guideline.

Completely aside from all the technological issues that need to be resolved, aside from changes that affect only one individual, and aside from whether possibilities such as discussed by Renee Wegrzyn in her 2017 LongNow talk (thanks, Hank!) become possible and it may become possible to undo germline modifications, I can imagine taking germ-line modifications forward very slowly and addressing conditions on the basis of their negative impact on life, namely specifically whether they allow an individual to mature to the age of majority or not.

Starting with the most serious conditions – the ones that currently mean that babies suffer terribly and die soon – harbors the smallest possibilities for harm and as much potential for learning and perfecting the technologies as is possible through other modifications. We owe that to these individuals.

Once we have learned how to deal with such conditions successfully, we can progressively work our way to all genetic conditions that stop people from reaching the age of majority. Again, we owe that to these individuals.

For some conditions, if we can't remedy them, we might consider introducing the FAAH-OUT gene mutation that stops people from feeling pain. If a Scottish pensioner can live to the age of 65 without knowing that she has this condition, it may have far fewer risks than I would have expected (as pain generally has a clear signaling function).

By that time, all or most concerns that we currently have should have dropped away and it should be allowed to tackle all other genetic disease-causing conditions, regardless of the question of whether I would personally like that or not. We will have to come up with a good definition of what is "disease-causing" and what is not, what should be "remedied" and whatnot, and a lot of the steering will have to come from the people who have certain conditions. We have to ask them what they want, not make assumptions such as that the lives of all different-bodied people are horrible.

So much will have changed by that time that I cannot possibly foresee what might be desirable or even moral by then and what wouldn't. Any current deliberations of what should and should not be considered "good health" and what treatments should and should not be available to everyone are by necessity hampered by their inability to include the future.

By that time, we will no longer be making our babies in uteruses and by that time, so much will have changed that, we will need to have (had) a new discussion about what kind of enhancements we want to allow and which ones we don't want. But at this point in time, we should not go there, simply because humans are not Gucci bags.

I hope that we will be able to change our skin tone in the morning, the way we now pick our clothes and that this will include colors like purple, blue and fluorescent green. We've already made "glow-in-the-dark" mammals (cats and mice) into which the inserted the genes of glow-in-the-dark fish species, so why not?

# Afterword

We'll also be integrated much more technology. We'll all be "biotech" combinations to a greater extent than the one "eyeborg" we currently have (Neil Harbisson) and who still gets kicked out of department stores because he looks different.

But before that, we will first need to save the planet because if we don't, we will soon cease to exist as a species.

Personally, I want a future in which animal abuse by humans no longer occurs because we have absolutely no justification for the horrors that we are currently inflicting on other sentient beings, many of which belong to species that have roamed the earth for many more years than we have. The fact that we humans still inflict similar horrors on members of our own species tells me that we have a long way to go. The current trends of emancipation provide a great deal of hope, however.

**We need to talk about this**

# 13. Sources of information

*"You cannot transmit wisdom and insight to another person. The seed is already there. A good teacher touches the seed, allowing it to wake up, to sprout, and to grow."*

– Thích Nhất Hạnh

### Articles in newspapers, magazines and on blogs

Adam, Betty Ann (2015) Saskatoon Health Region apologizes after aboriginal women felt pressured by staff to have tubes tied. Postmedia News. Published online on 17 November 2015. Available at http://news.nationalpost.com/news/canada/saskatoon-health-region-apologizes-after-aboriginal-women-felt-pressured-by-staff-to-have-tubes-tied

Agerholm, Harriet (2017) Japan urged to scrap law forcing transgender people to be sterilised before they can transition. The Independent. Published online on 1 December 2017. Available at http://www.independent.co.uk/news/world/asia/japan-transgender-people-sterilise-before-transition-gender-change-lgbt-rights-a8086341.html

Akwagyiram, Alexis (2004) Profiling the stalker and victim. BBC News Online. Available at http://news.bbc.co.uk/1/hi/uk/3717696.stm

Alderson, Andrew, Leapman, Ben, and Harper, Tom. (2007) System taking hundreds of babies for adoption. The Telegraph. Published online on 1 July 2007. Available at http://www.telegraph.co.uk/news/uknews/1556114/System-taking-hundreds-of-babies-for-adoption.html

Alston, Philip (2018) Statement on Visit to the United Kingdom, by Professor Philip Alston, United Nations Special Rapporteur on extreme poverty and human rights. Published on 16 November 2018. Available at https://www.ohchr.org/Documents/Issues/Poverty/EOM_GB_16Nov2018.pdf

Andersen, Ross. (2012) Why cognitive enhancement is in your future (and your past) (an interview with Allen Buchanan), The Atlantic, February 6 issue. Available at https://www.theatlantic.com/technology/archive/2012/02/why-cognitive-enhancement-is-in-your-future-and-your-past/252566/

Aubry, Jason (2017) Ohio lawmakers hear bill that would criminalize aborting children with Down Syndrome. NBC4i. Published online on 24 August 2017. Available at http://nbc4i.com/2017/08/24/lawmakers-hear-bill-that-would-criminalize-aborting-children-with-down-syndrome/

BBC News (2017) Women 'should be told' sex of foetus in pregnancy scan. BBC News. March 19 issue. Available at http://www.bbc.co.uk/news/uk-39319537

Baylis, Françoise (2017) Human genome editing: We should all have a say. The Conversation. Published online on 2 August 2017. Available at https://theconversation.com/human-genome-editing-we-should-all-have-a-say-81797

Baynes, Chris (2018) Japanese woman forcibly sterilised as teenager suing government for breach of human rights. The Independent. Published online on 1 February 2018. Available at http://www.independent.co.uk/news/world/asia/japanese-woman-forcibly-sterilised-teenager-15-suing-government-human-rights-a8188351.html?S2ref=549379

BBC (2019) Dalian Atkinson: Police officer charged with footballer murder. BBC News. Published online on 7 November 2019. Available at https://www.bbc.co.uk/news/uk-england-50333081

Beals, Daniel (2005) The Groningen Protocol: Making infanticide legal does not make it moral. The Center for Ethics & Human Dignity, Trinity University. Published online on 23 March 2005. Available at https://cbhd.org/content/groningen-protocol-making-infanticide-legal-does-not-make-it-moral

Begley, Sharon (2017) 5 things to know about the experimental treatment Charlie Gard might receive. STAT. Published online on 17 July 2017. Available at https://www.statnews.com/2017/07/17/charlie-gard-treatment/

# Sources of information

Bikwas, Soutik (2014) India's dark history of sterilization. BBC News. Published online on November 14. Available at http://www.bbc.co.uk/news/world-asia-india-30040790

Bindel, Julie (2005) The life stealers. The Guardian. Published online on 16 April 2005. Available at https://www.theguardian.com/uk/2005/apr/16/ukcrime.weekend7

Bowcott, Owen (2014) Mother who drank heavily when pregnant not guilty of crime, court rules. The Guardian. Published online on 4 December 2014. Available at https://www.theguardian.com/law/2014/dec/04/mother-drank-heavily-pregnant-not-guilty-crime

Bradley Hagerty, Barbara (2017) When Your Child Is a Psychopath. The Atlantic. Published online in June 2017. Available at https://www.theatlantic.com/magazine/archive/2017/06/when-your-child-is-a-psychopath/524502/

Burke, Jason (2014) India mass sterilisation: women were 'forced' into camps, say relatives. The Guardian. Published online on 12 November 2014. Available at https://www.theguardian.com/world/2014/nov/12/india-sterilisation-deaths-women-forced-camps-relatives

Burke, Kevin (2017) Disappearance of Down syndrome children in Iceland reveals the slippery slope of prenatal testing to abortion. Washington Examiner. Published online on 16 August 2017. Available at http://www.washingtonexaminer.com/disappearance-of-down-syndrome-children-in-iceland-reveals-the-slippery-slope-of-prenatal-testing-to-abortion/article/2631689

Cassidy, John (2018) 'Shopping can be so embarrassing for me'. Business reporter, BBC News. Published online on 13 November 2018. Available at https://www.bbc.co.uk/news/business-46155498

CBC News (2013) Halifax mom questions Down syndrome suppression. CBC News. Published online on 23 July 2013. Available at http://www.cbc.ca/beta/news/canada/nova-scotia/halifax-mom-questions-down-syndrome-suppression-1.1323401

Chicago Tribune (1997) Europe's taboo, sterilization, out of shadows. Chicago Tribune, issue of 28 August 1997. Available at http://articles.chicagotribune.com/1997-08-28/news/9708280294_1_sterilizations-handicapped-nazi-dictator-adolf-hitler

Cohen, I. Glenn (2017) Artificial wombs and abortion rights. DOI: 10.1002/hast.730

Cohen, Jon (2016) Stopping CRISPR's genome-editing scissors from snipping out of control, Science. doi:10.1126/science.aal0491 Available at http://www.sciencemag.org/news/2016/12/stopping-crispr-s-genome-editing-scissors-snipping-out-control

Cokley, Rebecca (2017) Please don't edit me out. Washington Post. Published online on 10 August 2017. Available at https://www.washingtonpost.com/opinions/if-we-start-editing-genes-people-like-me-might-not-exist/2017/08/10/e9adf206-7d27-11e7-a669-b400c5c7e1cc_story.html?utm_term=.964f93721b4b

Connor, Steve (2014) Three-parent babies: 'As long as she's healthy, I don't care', says mother of IVF child. The Independent. Published online on 25 August 2014. Available at http://www.independent.co.uk/news/science/three-child-babies-the-mothers-view-as-long-as-she-s-healthy-i-don-t-care-9690059.html

Cook-Degan, Robert and Maienschein, Jane (2017) Listening for the public voice. Discussions about genetic engineering in humans need input from nonexperts. Slate. Available at http://www.slate.com/articles/technology/future_tense/2017/08/the_public_needs_to_weigh_in_on_the_ethics_of_genetically_engineering_humans.html

Cowen, Tyler (2017)The Drive for Perfect Children Gets a Little Scary. Bloomberg, Published online on 24 August 2017. Available at https://www.bloomberg.com/view/articles/2017-08-24/the-drive-for-perfect-children-gets-a-little-scary

Cyranoski, David (2017) China's embrace of embryo selection raises thorny questions. Nature 548, 272-274. doi:10.1038/548272a Available at http://www.nature.com/news/china-s-embrace-of-embryo-selection-raises-thorny-questions-1.22468

Davies, Caroline (2017) Charlie Gard's short life pitched parents into turmoil and grief The Guardian. Published online on 28 July 2017. Available at https://www.theguardian.com/uk-news/2017/jul/28/charlie-gards-short-life-pitched-parents-into-turmoil-and-grief

Davies, Sally (2013) Encounters with the posthuman. Nautilus. Published online on April 29 2013. Available at http://nautil.us/issue/1/what-makes-you-so-special/encounters-with-the-posthuman

Davis, Nicola (2020) Long-term offenders have different brain structure, study says. The Guardian. First published online Mon 17 Feb 2020 23.30 GMT, last modified on Tue 18 Feb 2020 00.25 GMT. Available at https://www.theguardian.com/science/2020/feb/17/long-term-offenders-have-different-brain-structure-study-says

Dreger, Alice (2013) For kids, plastic surgery not always the answer. The Atlantic, May 21 issue. Available at https://www.theatlantic.com/health/archive/2013/05/for-kids-plastic-surgery-not-always-the-answer/276077/

Edwards, Jessica (2019) Age-related immaturity in the classroom can lead to ADHD misdiagnosis. Published online in December 2019. Available at https://www.acamh.org/research-digests/age-immaturity-classroom-adhd-misdiagnosis/

Elgot, Jessica (2013) Italian woman Alessandra Pacchieri calls on U.K. Social Service to return 'forced caesarean' baby. The Huffington Post. Published online on 5 December 2013; updated on 23 January 2014. Available at http://www.huffingtonpost.co.uk/2013/12/05/italy-forced-caesarean_n_4388894.html

Elgot, Jessica (2015) Blind man Tasered by police paid undisclosed sum. The Guardian. Published online on Thu 20 Aug 2015 13.13 BST. Last modified on Thu 21 Sep 2017 00.32 BST. Available at https://www.theguardian.com/uk-news/2015/aug/20/blind-man-tasered-by-police-paid-undisclosed-sumwhite-stick-samurai-sword

Emmerich, Nathan (2013) Bioethicists must not allow themselves to become a 'priestly caste'. The increasing use of expert bioethicists has profound anti-democratic implications. The Guardian. Published online on 14 May 2013. Available at https://www.theguardian.com/science/political-science/2013/may/14/bioethicists-priestly-caste

Florida Center for Instructional Technology (1997-2013) A teacher's guide to the Holocaust. Florida Center for Instructional Technology, College of Education, University of South Florida. Available at https://fcit.usf.edu/holocaust/people/victims.htm

Friedersdorf, Conor (2015) Methods That Police Use on the Mentally Ill Are Madness. The Atlantic. Available at https://www.theatlantic.com/politics/archive/2015/03/methods-that-cops-use-with-the-mentally-ill-are-madness/388610/

Galeon, Dom, and Reedy, Christianna (2017) Kurzweil Claims That the Singularity Will Happen by 2045. Futurism. Available at https://futurism.com/kurzweil-claims-that-the-singularity-will-happen-by-2045/

Gregory, Andy (2020) Jonty Bravery: Tate Modern attacker 'told carers of plan to kill stranger'. The Independent. Published online on 7 February 2020. Available at https://www.independent.co.uk/news/uk/crime/tate-modern-attack-boy-jonty-bravery-plan-recorded-tape-carers-a9322841.html

Guardian, The (2018) Anatomy of a police shooting: the final hours of Elijah Holcombe. The Guardian. Published online on Sun 27 May 2018 19.00 BST. Available at https://www.theguardian.com/australia-news/2018/may/28/anatomy-of-a-police-shooting-the-final-hours-of-elijah-holcombe (See also https://www.smh.com.au/national/nsw/elijah-holcombe-not-a-threat-when-shot-by-police-coroner-20140501-37k3j.html and https://www.abc.net.au/7.30/elijah-holcombes-inquest-resumes/4593678 and https://www.smh.com.au/entertainment/books/waiting-for-elijah-a-tragedy-that-didn-t-have-to-happen-20180606-p4zjri.html)

Hargreaves, Adam (2017) Introducing 'dark DNA' – the phenomenon that could change how we think about evolution. The Conversation. Published online on 24 August 2017. Available at https://theconversation.com/introducing-dark-dna-the-phenomenon-that-could-change-how-we-think-about-evolution-82867

Harper, Joyce (in cooperation with Bawden, Tom) (2017) Scientists call for new rules on GM designer babies. Inews. Available online at https://inews.co.uk/news/health/new-rules-will-be-needed-to-exploit-designer-baby-breakthrough-in-britain/

Harris, John (2020) Locked away: the national scandal you may have missed. The Guardian. Published online on 17 February 2020 at 06.00 GMT. Available at https://www.theguardian.com/commentisfree/2020/feb/17/national-scandal-nhs-local-authorities-vulnerable-people

Hayward, Charlotte (2019) 'We were bullied out of our home for being different' BBC News. Published online on 6 May 2019. Available at https://www.bbc.co.uk/news/stories-48154578

Hesman Saey, Tina (2017) Gene editing of human embryos gets rid of a mutation that causes heart failure. Success in correcting DNA defect inches use of CRISPR closer to clinical trial. Science 192 (3), 6. Available at https://www.sciencenews.org/article/crispr-gene-editing-human-embryos

Houser, Kristin (2019) China quietly confirms birth of third gene-edited baby. Futurism. Published online on 30 December 2019. Available at https://futurism.com/neoscope/china-confirms-birth-third-gene-edited-baby

Human Fertilisation and Embryology Authority (2005) Choices & boundaries. Should people be able to select embryos free from an inherited susceptibility to cancer? Public consultation. HFEA. Available at http://hfeaarchive.uksouth.cloudapp.azure.com/www.hfea.gov.uk/docs/Choices_and_Boundaries.pdf

Hunter, Philip (2010) The psycho gene. EMBO reports 11(9), 667-669. doi:10.1038/embor.2010.122 Available at https://www.ncbi.nlm.nih.gov/pmc/articles/PMC2933872/

Inquest (2018) Police misconduct hearing following death of Kingsley Burrell to conclude. Inquest. Published online on 14 December 2018. Available at https://www.inquest.org.uk/kingsley-burrell-misconduct-conclusion

International Initiative for Mental Health Leadership (2016) The use of Tasers on people with mental health problems across IIMHL countries. IIMHL. Published online in October 2016. Available at http://www.iimhl.com/files/docs/Make_It_So/20161020.pdf

Jabour, Bridie (2015) UN examines Australia's forced sterilisation of women with disabilities. The Guardian. Published online on 10 November 2015; last modified on 26 October 2016. Available at https://www.theguardian.com/australia-news/2015/nov/10/un-examines-australias-forced-sterilisation-of-women-with-disabilities

Jha, Alok (2011) Glow cat: fluorescent green felines could help study of HIV. The Guardian. Published online on 11 September 2011. Available at https://www.theguardian.com/science/2011/sep/11/genetically-modified-glowing-cats

Joncour, Nicolas (2016) The right to an education. Website of Henny Kupferstein. Available at https://hennyk.com/2016/09/26/the-right-to-an-education-article-typed-by-non-verbal-autistic-piano-student-with-dyspraxia/

Kentish, Benjamin (2018) MPs approve 'Seni's law' to restrict use of force against mental health patients. The Independent. Published online at Friday 6 July 2018 13:58. Available at https://www.independent.co.uk/news/uk/politics/senis-law-olaseni-lewis-mental-health-uk-government-mps-patients-a8435161.html

Kickbusch, Ilona (2020) The dark side of digital health. BMJ blog. Published on 14 January 2020. Available at https://blogs.bmj.com/bmj/2020/01/14/ilona-kickbusch-the-dark-side-of-digital-health/

King, David (2017) Editing the human genome brings us one step closer to consumer eugenics. The Guardian. Published online on 4 August 2017. Available at https://www.theguardian.com/commentisfree/2017/aug/04/editing-human-genome-consumer-eugenics-designer-babies

## Sources of information

Klosterman, Chuck (2013) There are no sound moral arguments against performance-enhancing drugs. The Ethicist (The New York Times Magazine). Published online on August 30. Available at http://www.nytimes.com/2013/09/01/magazine/there-are-no-sound-moral-arguments-against-performance-enhancing-drugs.html

Ko, Lisa (2016) Unwanted sterilization and eugenics programs in the United States. PBS, Human Rights Section. Published online on January 29, 2016. Available at http://www.pbs.org/independentlens/blog/unwanted-sterilization-and-eugenics-programs-in-the-united-states/

Kuiper, Martin and Weeda, Frederiek (2010) Politie sluit nog vaak verwarde mensen op (Dutch). NRC. Published online on 7 January 2020. Available at https://www.nrc.nl/nieuws/2020/01/07/politie-sluit-nog-vaak-verwarde-mensen-op-a3986049

Kula, Shane (2016) Three-Parent Children Are Already Here. In the late '90s and early '00s, 30 to 50 children were born using techniques similar to those under debate now. Slate. Published online on 18 February 2016. Available at http://www.slate.com/articles/technology/future_tense/2016/02/three_parent_babies_have_been_here_since_the_late_90s.html

Lant, Karla, and Norman, Abby (2017) Tech expert warns that AI could become "a fascist's dream". Futurism. Available at https://futurism.com/tech-expert-warns-that-ai-could-become-a-fascists-dream/

Ledford, Heidi (2016) CRISPR: gene editing is just the beginning. Nature 531, 156-159. Available at http://www.nature.com/news/crispr-gene-editing-is-just-the-beginning-1.19510

Lizarzaburu, Javier (2015) Forced sterilisation haunts Peruvian women decades on. BBC News. Published online on December 2, 2015. Available at http://www.bbc.co.uk/news/world-latin-america-34855804

MacAttram, Matilda (2016) Tasers have no place in mental health care. The Guardian. Published on Mon 18 Jul 2016 15.15 BSTLast modified on Wed 20 Sep 2017 19.21 BST .Available at https://www.theguardian.com/healthcare-network/2016/jul/18/tasers-have-no-place-in-mental-health-care

Marsh, Sarah, Dodd, Vikram and Grierson, Jamie (2019) Police chiefs criticise £10m Taser rollout. The Guardian. Published online on Fri 27 Sep 2019 at 16.08 BST. Available at https://theguardian.com/uk-news/2019/sep/27/police-in-england-and-wales-to-be-given-more-tasers-in-10m-rollout

Mason, Rowena and Sample, Ian (2020) Sabisky row: Dominic Cummings criticised over 'designer babies' post. The Guardian. Published online at 19:06 on 19 February 2020. Available at https://www.theguardian.com/politics/2020/feb/19/sabisky-row-dominic-cummings-criticised-over-designer-babies-post

MacKinnon, J.B. (2018) It's Tough Being a Right Whale These Days. The Atlantic. Published online on 30 July2018.

Mind (2017) PIP ruling a 'victory for people with mental health problems', says Mind. Mind. Published online on 21 December 2017. Available at https://www.mind.org.uk/news-campaigns/news/pip-ruling-a-victory-for-people-with-mental-health-problems-says-mind/#.WnGRgdRpH3A

Morris, Steven (2018) Bristol man with autism shot by police with stun gun. The Guardian. Published online on Wed 31 Jan 2018 11.19 GMT Last modified on Wed 31 Jan 2018 22.00 GMT. Available at https://www.theguardian.com/uk-news/2018/jan/31/bristol-man-with-autism-shot-by-police-with-stun-gun

Morris, Steven (2019) Police disciplinary hearings dropped over Thomas Orchard death. The Guardian. Published online on Thu 24 Oct 2019 16.03 BST. Last modified on Thu 24 Oct 2019 19.50 BST. Available at https://www.theguardian.com/uk-news/2019/oct/24/disciplinary-hearings-dropped-over-thomas-orchards-death

Nelson, Fraser (2016) The return of eugenics. The Spectator, April 2 issue. Available at https://www.spectator.co.uk/2016/04/the-return-of-eugenics/

Ohikuare, Judith (2014) Life as a nonviolent psychopath. The Atlantic, January 21 issue. Available at http://www.theatlantic.com/health/archive/2014/01/life-as-a-nonviolent-psychopath/282271/

Oosterom, Rianne (2017) Woede over taseren patiënt in isoleercel (Dutch). Trouw. Published online on 5 September 2017 at 18:11. Available at https://www.trouw.nl/samenleving/woede-over-taseren-patient-in-isoleercel~a420b81a/

Paris, J.J., Ahluwalia, J., Cummings, BM, Moreland, MP, and Wilkinson, D.J. (2017) The Charlie Gard case: British and American approaches to court resolution of disputes over medical decisions. Journal of Perinatology 37(12), 1269-1271. Available at https://www.ncbi.nlm.nih.gov/pmc/articles/PMC5712473/

Potter, Jessica (2017) New discriminatory NHS policy is bad for your health, whoever you are. The Conversation. Published online on 29 September 2017. Available at https://theconversation.com/new-discriminatory-nhs-policy-is-bad-for-your-health-whoever-you-are-84855

Potter, Jessica (2017) NHS urged to share data so patients can be deported. Published online on 6 February 2017. Available at https://theconversation.com/nhs-urged-to-share-data-so-patients-can-be-deported-72380

Pressman, Matthew (2013) The Myth of FDR's Secret Disability. Time. Published online on July 12, 2013. Available at http://ideas.time.com/2013/07/12/the-myth-of-fdrs-secret-disability/

Radio Sweden (2012) ADHD diagnosis "may just reflect immaturity". Radio Sweden. Published online on 10 May 2012. Available at: https://sverigesradio.se/sida/artikel.aspx?programid=2054&artikel=5101644

Rawlinson, Kevin and Adams, Richard (2018) UCL to investigate eugenics conference secretly held on campus. The Guardian. Published online on 11 January 2018. Available at https://www.theguardian.com/education/2018/jan/10/ucl-to-investigate-secret-eugenics-conference-held-on-campus

Regalado, Antonio (2015) Engineering the perfect baby. MIT Technology Review. Published online on 5 March 2015. Available at https://www.technologyreview.com/s/535661/engineering-the-perfect-baby/

Regalado, Antonio (2016) Human-animal chimeras are gestating on U.S. research farms. MIT Technology Review. Published online on 6 January 2016. Available at https://www.technologyreview.com/s/545106/human-animal-chimeras-are-gestating-on-us-research-farms/

Regalado, Antonio (2017) Doctors plan bold test of gene therapy on boys with muscular dystrophy. MIT Technology Review. Published online on 17 August 2017. Available at https://www.technologyreview.com/s/608575/doctors-plan-bold-test-of-gene-therapy-on-boys-with-muscular-dystrophy/

Reuell, Peter (2017) New insight on height, arthritis. Harvard Gazette, 25 July. Available at https://news.harvard.edu/gazette/story/2017/07/new-insight-on-height-arthritis

Reuters (2017) Inside the Taser, the weapon that transformed policing. Shock Tactics. Reuters Investigates. Available at https://www.reuters.com/investigates/section/usa-taser/

Robins, Jon (2015) Majority of suspects Tasered by police are mentally ill, figures show. The Independent. Published online on Saturday 26 December 2015 23:25. Available at http://www.independent.co.uk/news/uk/crime/majority-of-suspects-tasered-by-police-are-mentally-ill-figures-show-a6786996.html

Rochman, Bonnie (2017) The disturbing, eugenics-like reality unfolding in Iceland. Quartz. Published online on 19 August 2017. Available at https://qz.com/1056810/the-disturbing-eugenics-like-reality-unfolding-in-iceland/

RTE (2017) Jaarverslag 2018. RTE. 31 pages. Available at https://www.euthanasiecommissie.nl/de-toetsingscommissies/uitspraken/jaarverslagen/2016/april/12/jaarverslag-2016

## Sources of information

RTL (2017) Patiënt getaserd in isoleercel: 'onmenselijke behandeling', zegt Amnesty International (Dutch). RTL Nieuws. Published online on 05 September 2017 16:12. Adapted on 13 November 2017 20:10. Available online at https://www.rtlnieuws.nl/nederland/artikel/2590131/patient-getaserd-isoleercel-onmenselijke-behandeling-zegt-amnesty

Rucke, Katie (2013) Five Texas Police Departments Ban Tasers. Mint Press News. Published online on 26 September 2013. Available at https://www.mintpressnews.com/five-texas-police-departments-ban-tasers/169669/

Rutecki, Gregory W. (2010) Forced sterilization of Native Americans: Late twentieth century physician cooperation with national eugenic policies. The Center for Bioethics and Human Dignity, Trinity International University. Published online on October 8, 2010. Available at https://cbhd.org/content/forced-sterilization-native-americans-late-twentieth-century-physician-cooperation-national-

Saini, Angela (2020) Eugenics refuses to die – and now Andrew Sabisky has put it back in the headlines. The Guardian. Published online at 11:07 on 19 February 2020. Available at https://www.theguardian.com/commentisfree/2020/feb/19/eugenics-andrew-sabisky-right-ideas-human-breeding

Salman, Saba (2018) What would a truly disabled-accessible city look like? The Guardian. Published online on 14 February 2018. Available at https://www.theguardian.com/cities/2018/feb/14/what-disability-accessible-city-look-like

Salter, Frank K. (2015) Eugenics, ready or not. Quadrant. Published online on 11 May 2015. Available at https://quadrant.org.au/magazine/2015/05/eugenics-ready/

Sandel, Michael J. (2004) The Case Against Perfection, The Atlantic, April issue. Available at https://www.theatlantic.com/magazine/archive/2004/04/the-case-against-perfection/302927/

Satoshi, Fukuma (2011) Fit for the Future? Modern technology, liberal democracy and the urgent need for moral improvement, in: DALS Newsletter 28/29, page 14. Available at http://www.l.u-tokyo.ac.jp/shiseigaku/pdf/NL28-29e.pdf

Saul, Heather (2016) Professor Stephen Hawking: Humanity will not survive another 1,000 years if we don't escape our planet. The Independent. Published online on 15 November 2016. Available at http://www.independent.co.uk/news/people/professor-stephen-hawking-humanity-wont-survive-1000-years-on-earth-a7417366.html

Schmitt, David P. (2016) Sex and Gender Are Dials (Not Switches). Sexual diversity as obliquely interconnected dimensions. Psychology Today. Published online 13 May 2016. Available at https://www.psychologytoday.com/blog/sexual-personalities/201605/sex-and-gender-are-dials-not-switches

Scottish Council on Human Bioethics (2006) Response to HFEA consultation "Choices & boundaries. Should people be able to select embryos free from an inherited susceptibility to cancer?" SCHB. Available at http://www.schb.org.uk/downloads/publications/consult_choices_and_boundaries_jan06.pdf

Shaw. Danny (2019) PTSD 'at crisis levels' among police officers. BBC News. Published online on 9 May 2019. Available at https://www.bbc.co.uk/news/uk-48201088

Smith, Jennifer and Osborne, Lucy (2014) Man who died after being Tasered by police was 'not breaking into flats but visiting friends for birthday drink'. Published online: 12:05, 25 December 2014 | Updated: 15:35, 25 December 2014. Available at https://www.dailymail.co.uk/news/article-2886925/Man-died-Tasered-police-reports-break-block-flats-visiting-friends-quiet-birthday-drink.html

Stromberg, Joseph (2013) The neuroscientist who discovered he was a psychopath. smithsonian.com. Published online on November 22, 2013. Available at http://www.smithsonianmag.com/science-nature/the-neuroscientist-who-discovered-he-was-a-psychopath-180947814/

Smith, David (2018) Ex-tech workers plead with Facebook: consider the harm you are doing to kids. The Guardian. Published online on 8 February 2018. Available at https://www.theguardian.com/technology/2018/feb/07/facebook-common-sense-media-tech-addictions-children

# Sources of information

Stuff (2017) Police use of Taser on mentally-ill man ruled as excessive and unjustified. Stuff. Published online on Mar 09 2017 at 11:19. Available at http://www.stuff.co.nz/national/crime/90230066/Police-use-of-Taser-on-mentally-ill-man-ruled-as-excessive-and-unjustified

The Economist (1997) Nordic eugenics. Here, of all places. The Economist, Issue of August 28 1997. Available at http://www.economist.com/node/155244

Thomasen, Katrine (2016) Advancing women's sexual and reproductive rights in Europe – a snapshot of legal and policy progress from 1986 to 2016. WHO. Available at http://www.euro.who.int/__data/assets/pdf_file/0015/330090/4-Advancing-womens-sexual-reproductive-rights-in-Europe.pdf

Tingley, Kim (2014) The Brave New World of Three-Parent I.V.F. New York Times. Published online on 27 June 2014. Accessible at https://www.nytimes.com/2014/06/29/magazine/the-brave-new-world-of-three-parent-ivf.html

Tremonti, Anna Maria, and Mattar, Pacinthe (2016) Aboriginal women say they were sterilized against their will in hospital. CBC. Published online on January 7. Available at http://www.cbc.ca/radio/thecurrent/the-current-for-january-7-2016-1.3393099/aboriginal-women-say-they-were-sterilized-against-their-will-in-hospital-1.3393143

Walsh, Fergus (2020) Gene therapy to halt rare form of sight loss. BBC. Published online on 17 February 2020. Available at https://www.bbc.co.uk/news/health-51533922

WHO (2017) "Depression: let's talk" says WHO, as depression tops list of causes of ill health. News release. WHO. Published online 30 March 2017. Available at http://www.who.int/mediacentre/news/releases/2017/world-health-day/en/

Wilkinson, Dominic and Savulescu, Julian (2017) Hard lessons: learning from the Charlie Gard case. Practical Ethics. Published online on 24 July 2017. Available at http://blog.practicalethics.ox.ac.uk/2017/07/hard-lessons-learning-from-the-charlie-gard-case/

Young Minds (2018) Victory For Campaigners as Seni's Law Passes. Young Minds. Published online on 01 November 2018. Available at https://youngminds.org.uk/blog/victory-for-campaigners-as-seni-s-law-passes/

**Books and book chapters**

Bintanja, Richard (2017) The ultimate brainchild. Marisuda, Lelystad, the Netherlands. 227 pages. (English translation by Angelina Souren of Dutch original.) ISBN/EAN 978-90-818264-3-3. (Also available as e-book.)

Buchanan, Allen (2013) Beyond humanity?: The ethics of biomedical enhancement. Oxford University Press. 298 pages.

Coelho, Paulo (2008) The winner stands alone. Translated from the Portuguese by Margaret Jull Costa. HarperCollinsPublishers. 373 pages.

Connolly, Joseph (2015) Style. Quercus, London, U.K. 489 pages.

Fieser, James (2001) Moral philosophy through the ages. McGraw-Hill Higher Education. 294 pages. The chapter on utilitarianism can be accessed at https://www.utm.edu/staff/jfieser/class/300/utilitarian.htm

Harris, John (2016) How to be good. Oxford University Press. 224 pages.

Kuhse, Helga, Schuklenk, Udo, and Singer, Peter (Editors) (2015) Bioethics: An Anthology, 3rd Edition. Wiley-Blackwell. 800 pages.

Persson, Ingmar, and Savulescu, Julian (2012) Unfit for the future. Oxford University Press. 156 pages.

Sandel, Michael J. (2009) Justice. What's the right thing to do? Penguin Books, 308 pages.

Sandel, Michael (2009) The case against perfection. Harvard University Press. 176 pages.

Unger, David (2011) Chapter 5: Genetic and reproductive control. In: The Canadian bioethics companion. an online textbook for Canadian ethicists and health care workers. Available at http://canadianbioethicscompanion.ca/the-canadian-bioethics-companion/chapter-5-genetic-and-reproductive-control/

Wilkinson, Dominic (2016) Chapter 4 Who should decide for critically ill neonates and how? The grey zone in neonatal treatment decisions. In: McDougall R, Delany C, Gillam L, editors. When Doctors and Parents Disagree: Ethics, Paediatrics & the Zone of Parental Discretion. The Federation Press, Sydney, Australia. 13 pages. Available at https://www.ncbi.nlm.nih.gov/pubmed/28661627

Wilson, E.O. (2016) Half-Earth: Our Planet's Fight for Life. Liveright, New York, U.S.A. 272 pages.

**Courses**

Cohen, I. Glenn and others. EDX course "Bioethics: The Law, Medicine, and Ethics of Reproductive Technologies and Genetics. An introduction to the study of bioethics and the application of legal and ethical reasoning." by Harvard Law School.

https://www.edx.org/course/bioethics-law-medicine-ethics-harvardx-hls4x-0

Amnesty International, Curtin University, Louvain University and others. Human rights courses on EDX
https://www.edx.org/course?search_query=human+rights

Sandel, Michael J. EDX course "Justice. What's the right thing to do?" by Harvard University.
https://www.youtube.com/watch?v=kBdfcR-8hEY&list=PL30C13C91CFFEFEA6
https://www.edx.org/course/justice-harvardx-er22-1x-2

Souren, Angelina. Bioethics, the ethics of everyday life.
https://www.udemy.com/course/bioethics-the-ethics-of-everyday-life/

Unesco. Climate Justice: Lessons from the Global South. Understand how we can balance human needs with caring for the planet with this free online course about climate change.
https://www.futurelearn.com/courses/climate-justice

University of Colorado, University of Strathclyde, University of New South Wales and others. Human rights courses on FutureLearn.
https://www.futurelearn.com/search?utf8=%E2%9C%93&q=human+rights

University of Michigan, University of Capetown, MIT and others. Justice courses on study.com.
https://study.com/articles/List_of_Free_Online_Criminal_Justice_Courses_Classes_and_Training_Programs.html

University of Sheffield, University of York, University of East Anglia and others. Justice courses on FutureLearn.
https://www.futurelearn.com/search?utf8=%E2%9C%93&q=justice

University of Twente. Philosophy of Technology and Design: Shaping the Relations Between Humans and Technologies.
https://www.futurelearn.com/courses/philosophy-of-technology

VanRooyen, Michael, Leaning, Jennifer and others (2016) EDX course "Humanitarian response to conflict and disaster" by Harvard Humanitarian Initiative and Harvard Center for Health and Human Rights.
https://www.edx.org/course/humanitarian-response-conflict-disaster-harvardx-ph558x-0

## Scholarly articles and reports

Alston, Philip (2019) Visit to the United Kingdom of Great Britain and Northern Ireland. Report of the Special Rapporteur on extreme poverty and human rights. A/HRC/41/39/Add.1. United Nations. Published on 23 April 2019.

Alston, Philip (2019) Report of the Special Rapporteur on extreme poverty and human rights. A/74/493. United Nations. Available at https://undocs.org/A/74/493 11 Oct 2019

Benston, Shawna (2016) CRISPR, a crossroads in genetic intervention: pitting the right to health against the right to disability. Laws 5(5); doi:10.3390/laws5010005. Available at http://www.mdpi.com/2075-471X/5/1/5/pdf

Bioethics Observatory (2017) The biological status of the early human embryo. When does human life begin? Bioethics Observatory - Institute of Life Sciences UCV. Published online on 13 June 2017. 14 pages. Available at http://www.bioethicsobservatory.org/2017/06/biological-status-early-human-embryo/21605

Boon, J.C.W. and Sheridan, L. (2001). Stalker typologies: A law enforcement perspective. Journal of Threat Assessment, 1, 75-97. (Can also be found in book published in May 2008: Stalking and Psychosexual Obsession: Psychological Perspectives for Prevention, Policing and Treatment, pages 63 - 82.) Available at https://www.researchgate.net/publication/227990165_Stalker_Typologies_Implications_for_Law_Enforcement

Brunetta d'Usseaux, Francesca (2001) Wrongful life and wrongful birth cases: a comparative approach. Etica & Politica / Ethics & Politics III (2001)1. 5 pages. Available at https://www.openstarts.units.it/handle/10077/5603

Buchanan-Smith, Maggie (2003) How the Sphere Project Came into Being: A Case Study of Policy-Making in the Humanitarian Aid Sector and the Relative Influence of Research. Working Paper 215. Overseas Development Institute, London, U.K. 34 pages.

Buiting, H.M., Karelse, M.A., Brouwers, H.A., Onwuteaka-Philipsen, B.D., Heide, A. van der, and Delden, J.J. van (2010) Dutch experience of monitoring active ending of life for newborns. J. Med Ethics 36(4), 234-237.

Cohen, Glenn I. (2009) Intentional diminishment, the non-identity problem, and legal liability. Hastings Law Journal 60: 347-375. Available at http://ssrn.com/abstract=1330504

Cohen, I Glenn and Chen, Daniel L. (2010) Trading-off reproductive technology and adoption: Does subsidizing IVF decrease adoption rates and should it matter? Minnesota Law Review 95, 485-577. Available at http://scholarship.law.duke.edu/cgi/viewcontent.cgi?article=2960&context=faculty_scholarship and https://papers.ssrn.com/sol3/papers.cfm?abstract_id=1664501

Cohen, I. Glenn, Savulescu, Julian, Adashi, Eli Y. (2015) Transatlantic lessons in regulation of mitochondrial replacement therapy. Science 348(6231), 178-180.

Condic, Maureen (2014) A Scientific View of When Life Begins. "On point" report by the Lozier Institute. 5 pages. Available at https://lozierinstitute.org/a-scientific-view-of-when-life-begins/

El-Toukhy, Tarek., Williams, Clare. and Braude Peter (2008) The ethics of preimplantation genetic diagnosis. The Obstetrician & Gynaecologist. doi:10.1576/toag.10.1.049.27378 Available at http://onlinelibrary.wiley.com/doi/10.1576/toag.10.1.049.27378/full

European Parliament (2016) Adoption without consent. Update 2016. Study for the Peti Committee. Available at http://www.europarl.europa.eu/RegData/etudes/STUD/2016/556940/IPOL_STU(2016)556940_EN.pdf

Faden, Ruth and Powers, Madison (2014) Biotechnology, Justice and Health. Journal of Practical Ethics, Vol. 1(2). Available at https://papers.ssrn.com/sol3/papers.cfm?abstract_id=2463192

Falzon, Christopher (2014) Wrongful birth and wrongful life: legal and moral issues. Master's thesis. University of Malta, 130 pages. DOI: 10.13140/RG.2.1.2156.4649 Available at https://www.researchgate.net/publication/281372405_Wrongful_Life_Wrongful_Birth_-_Legal_and_Moral_Issues

Ferrari, Alize J., Charlson, Fiona J., Norman, Rosana E., Patten, Scott B., Freedman, Greg, Murray, Christopher J.L., Vos, Theo, and Whiteford, Harvey A. (2013) Burden of depressive disorders by country, sex, age, and year: findings from the Global Burden of Disease study 2010. PLOS Medicine 10(11), 1-12. Available at http://journals.plos.org/plosmedicine/article?id=10.1371/journal.pmed.1001547

Fordham, Brigham A. (2011) Disability and designer babies. Valparaiso University Law Review 45(4), 159-214. Available at http://scholar.valpo.edu/cgi/viewcontent.cgi?article=2219&context=vulr

Fox, Dov (2007) The illiberality of 'liberal eugenics'. Available at http://works.bepress.com/dov_fox/13 and http://ssrn.com/abstract=1072104

Galton, David J. and Galton, Clare J. (1998) Francis Galton: and eugenics today. Journal of Medical Ethics 24, 99-105. Available at https://www.ncbi.nlm.nih.gov/pmc/articles/PMC1377454/

Giesen, I. (2009) Of wrongful birth, wrongful life, comparative law and the politics of tort law systems. Tydskrif vir Heedendaagse Romeins-Hollandse Reg (THRHR) 72, 257-273. Available at https://papers.ssrn.com/sol3/papers.cfm?abstract_id=1424901

Giesen, Ivo (2012) The Use and Influence of Comparative Law in 'Wrongful Life' Cases. Utrecht Law Review 8(2), 35-54. doi: 10.1136/jme.28.2.63 Available at https://papers.ssrn.com/sol3/papers.cfm?abstract_id=2063503

Greely, Henry T. (2008) Remarks on human biological enhancement. Kansas Law Review 56, 1139-1157. Available at https://law.drupal.ku.edu/sites/law.drupal.ku.edu/files/docs/law_review/v56/05%20-Greely%20Remarks_Final.pdf

Hendriks, S., Dancet, E.A., Pelt, A.M. van, Hamer, G., and Repping S. (2015) Artificial gametes: a systematic review of biological progress towards clinical application. Hum Reprod Update, 21(3), 285-296. Available at https://www.ncbi.nlm.nih.gov/pubmed/25609401/

Hiam, Lucinda, Steele, Sarah, and McKee, Martin (2018) Creating a 'hostile environment for migrants': the British government's use of health service data to restrict immigration is a very bad idea. Health Economics, Policy and Law. Published online on 8 January 2018. https://doi.org/10.1017/S1744133117000251

Human Fertilisation and Embryology Authority (2019) Fertility treatment 2017: trends and figures. HFEA. Available online at https://www.hfea.gov.uk/media/2894/fertility-treatment-2017-trends-and-figures-may-2019.pdf

Im, Wooseok, Moon, Jangsup, Kim, Manho (2016) Applications of CRISPR/Cas9 for Gene Editing in Hereditary Movement Disorders. J Mov Disord 9(3), 136-143. Available at https://www.e-jmd.org/journal/view.php?doi=10.14802/jmd.16029

Inhorn, Marcia C., and Patrizio, Pasquale (2015) Infertility around the globe: new thinking on gender, reproductive technologies and global movements in the 21st century. Human Reproduction Update 21(4), 411-426. Advanced Access publication on March 22, 2015 doi:10.1093/humupd/dmv016. Available at https://academic.oup.com/humupd/article/21/4/411/683746/Infertility-around-the-globe-new-thinking-on

Jayakumar, Sri Vidhya (2009) Liability of a mother for prenatal negligence to her child: A case for equal parenthood. Paper presented in the National Conference on Gender Equity at work and Home. A key to National Development held on 9-10 Jan. 2009 at K.G. Somaiya College, Mumbai, India. 8 pages

Jellison, S.S., Roberts, W., Bowers, A., Combs, T., Beaman, J., Wayant, C., Vassar, M. (2019). Evaluation of spin in abstracts of papers in psychiatry and psychology journals. BMJ: Evidence-Based Medicine. Published Online First: 05 August 2019. doi: 10.1136/bmjebm-2019-111176

Kamm, Frances (2005) "Is there a problem with enhancement?" The American Journal of Bioethics 5(3), 8-14.

Kass, Leon (1998) The wisdom of repugnance: why we should ban the cloning of humans. Valparaiso University Law Review 32(2), 679-705. Available at http://scholar.valpo.edu/vulr/vol32/iss2/12

King, Jaime S. (2008) Duty to the unborn: a response to Smolensky. Hastings Law Journal 60, 377-395. Available at http://repository.uchastings.edu/faculty_scholarship/327

Lindeman, Hilde and Verkerk. Marian (2008) Ending the Life of a Newborn: The Groningen Protocol. The Hastings Center Report, January-February 2008 issue, 42-51.

Lolas, Fernando (2008) Bioethics and animal research. A personal perspective and a note on the contribution of Fritz Jahr. Biol Res 41, 119-123. Available at https://scielo.conicyt.cl/pdf/bres/v41n1/art13.pdf

Lysaught, M. Therese (2002) Wrongful Life? The Strange Case of Nicholas Perruche. Commonweal 129(22 March), 9-11. Available at http://ecommons.luc.edu/ips_facpubs/8/

Macklin, Ruth (2003) Dignity is a useless concept. British Medical Journal 327, 1419-1420. Available at https://www.ncbi.nlm.nih.gov/pmc/articles/PMC300789/

National Council on Disability (2008) Finding the gaps: A comparative analysis of disability laws in the United States to the United Nations Convention on the Rights of Persons with Disabilities (CRPD). Available at http://www.hpod.org/

Nys, H.F.L.and Dute, J.C.J. (2004) A wrongful existence in the Netherlands. J Med Ethics 30,393-394. doi: 10.1136/jme.2003.005215 Available at http://jme.bmj.com/content/30/4/393

Ouellette, Alicia (2008) Insult to injury: A disability-sensitive response to Smolensky's call for parental tort liability for preimplantation genetic interventions. Hastings Law Journal 60, 397-410. Available at https://papers.ssrn.com/sol3/papers.cfm?abstract_id=1273714

Owagage, Mpaata (2014) Wrongful life:An analysis of cross-jurisdictional approaches. Melismata 1(February), 1-33. Available at http://law.unimelb.edu.au/__data/assets/pdf_file/0008/1595501/MELISMATA-ISSUE11.pdf

Pera, Alessandra (2017) Wrongful Birth and Wrongful Life. Floodgate argument and the balancing of contrasting rights in courts law making. Presented at 7th World Congress on Family Law and Children's Rights, 5-7 June 2017, Dublin, Ireland. Available at https://iris.unipa.it/retrieve/handle/10447/235873/437360/WrongfulBirthandWrongfulLifeFooldgateArgumentBalancingofcontrastinginterests.pdf

Perry, Ronen (2008) It's a wonderful life. Cornell Law Review 93, 329-399. Available at https://papers.ssrn.com/sol3/Papers.cfm?abstract_id=977852

Persson, Ingmar and Savulescu, Julian (2016) Moral bioenhancement, freedom and reason. Neuroethics. Published online 9 July. DOI 10.1007/s12152-016-9268-5. Available at https://link.springer.com/article/10.1007/s12152-016-9268-5

Pierce, Jessica and Bekoff, Marc (2018) A Postzoo Future: Why Welfare Fails Animals in Zoos, Journal of Applied Animal Welfare Science, 21:sup1, 43-48, DOI:10.1080/10888705.2018.1513838

Präg, Patrick, and Mills, Melinda C. (2015) Assisted reproductive technology in Europe. Usage and regulation in the context of cross-border reproductive care. Families and Societies, Working Paper Series 43. Also Forthcoming as a chapter in the volume Childlessness in Europe. Patterns, Causes, and Contexts, edited by Michaela Kreyenfeld and Dirk Konietzka. Available at http://www.familiesandsocieties.eu/wp-content/uploads/2015/09/WP43PragMills2015.pdf

Royal Courts of Justice (2014) CP (A Child) v First-Tier Tribunal (Criminal Injuries Compensation) & Ors [2014] EWCA Civ 1554 (04 December 2014) Case No: C3/2014/0775. Available at http://www.bailii.org/ew/cases/EWCA/Civ/2014/1554.html

Roberts, Andrea L., Lyall, Kristen, Rich-Edwards, Janet W., Ascherio, Alberto, and Weisskopf, Marc G. (2016) Maternal exposure to intimate partner abuse before birth is associated with autism spectrum disorder in offspring. Autism, 20(1): 26–36. doi:10.1177/1362361314566049.

Royal Courts of Justice (2017) Neutral Citation Number: [2017] EWHC 3375 (Admin) Case No: CO/2496/2017. Available at http://www.bailii.org/ew/cases/EWHC/Admin/2017/3375.html

Savulescu, Julian (2001) Procreative beneficence: Why we should select the best children. Bioethics 15(5/6), 413-426. Available at http://onlinelibrary.wiley.com/doi/10.1111/1467-8519.00251/epdf

Sheldon, Tony (2005) Dutch Supreme Court backs damages for child for having been born. BMJ 330 (2 April). Available at http://www.bmj.com/content/330/7494/747.1

Sheridan, Lorraine (2002) Types of stalker. Presentation given on 12 September, 2002 at 16:00. eBulletin University of Leicester. Available at https://www.le.ac.uk/press/ebulletin/archive/speaker_sheridan.html

Silverberg, Agustín, Villar, Marcelo J., and Mesurado, Belén (2017) Euthanasia in critically ill neonates in Argentina. Medicina e Morale 5, 591-601.

Simpson, Bob (2017) A "we"'problem for bioethics and the social sciences : a response to Barbara Prainsack. Science, technology, and human values. Deposited in Durham Research Online on 18 September 2017. 13 pages. Available at http://dro.dur.ac.uk/22917/

Smajdor, Anna and Cutas, Daniela (2015) Artificial Gametes. Background paper. Nuffield Council on Bioethics. 21 pages. Available at http://nuffieldbioethics.org/wp-content/uploads/Background-paper-2016-Artificial-gametes.pdf

Smolensky, Kirsten Rabe (2008) Creating children with disabilities: parental tort liability for preimplantation genetic interventions. Arizona Legal Studies, Discussion Paper No. 08-15. Available at http://ssrn.com/abstract=1158631

Spratt, David and Dunlop, Ian (2019) Existential climate-related security risk: A scenario approach. Breakthrough – National Centre for Climate Restoration. Policy paper. Available at https://docs.wixstatic.com/ugd/148cb0_b2c0c79dc4344b279bcf2365336ff23b.pdf

Spriggs , M., and Savulescu, J. (2002) The Perruche judgment and the "right not to be born". J Med Ethics 28, 63-64. Available at http://jme.bmj.com/content/28/2/63

Stein, Michael Ashley (2004) Generalizing disability. Michigan Law Review 102, 1601-1617.

Stein, Michael Ashley and Stein, Penelope J.S. (2007) Beyond disability civil rights. Hastings Law Journal 58, 1203-1240. Available at https://papers.ssrn.com/sol3/papers.cfm?abstract_id=1552010

Tilley, Elizabeth, Earle, Sarah, Walmsley, Jan and Atkinson, Dorothy (2012) 'The Silence is roaring': sterilization, reproductive rights and women with intellectual disabilities. Disability and Society 27(3) 413-426. Available at http://oro.open.ac.uk/30719/2/Silence_is_roaring.pdf

United Nations, Department of Economic and Social Affairs, Population Division (2015). World Fertility Patterns 2015 – Data Booklet (ST/ESA/SER.A/370), 30 pages. Available at http://www.un.org/en/development/desa/population/publications/pdf/fertility/world-fertility-patterns-2015.pdf

Velasquez, M., Andre, C., Shanks, T., and Meyer, M. J. (1989) Calculating consequences: The utilitarian approach to ethics. Issues in Ethics 2(1) (Winter 1989). Available at https://www.scu.edu/ethics/ethics-resources/ethical-decision-making/calculating-consequences-the-utilitarian-approach/

Verhagen, Eduard and Sauer, Pieter J.J. (2005) The Groningen Protocol – Euthanasia in severely ill newborns. N Engl J Med 352, 959-962. Available at http://www.nejm.org/doi/full/10.1056/NEJMp058026

Wijngaarden, Els van, Leget, Carlo and Goossensen, Anne (2015) Ready to give up on life: The lived experience of elderly people who feel life is completed and no longer worth living. Social Science & Medicine 138, 257-264. Available at https://ac.els-cdn.com/S0277953615002889/1-s2.0-S0277953615002889-main.pdf?_tid=80f432e0-edcd-11e7-993c-00000aab0f26&acdnat=1514685434_0b38f23b28ec70c2cd53776218c61c43

Wilkinson, James E. (2009) Groningen Protocol. Position Paper on the Disability Stereotypes, International Human Rights and Infanticide. International Federation for Spina Bifida and Hydrocephalus. Available at https://www.ifglobal.org/images/stories/groningen-d.pdf

Wilkinson, Dominic, Skene, Loane, Crespigny, Lachlan De, and Savulescu, Julian (2016) Protecting future children from in-utero harm. Bioethics 30(6), 425-432. doi:10.1111/bioe.12238 Available at https://www.ncbi.nlm.nih.gov/pmc/articles/PMC4913745/pdf/BIOE-30-425.pdf

**Videos**

Anholt, Simon. Which country does the most good for the world? https://www.ted.com/talks/simon_anholt_which_country_does_the_most_good_for_the_world

## Sources of information

Bohorquez, Diego. TED Talk: How does our gut talk to our brain?
https://www.youtube.com/watch?v=utFG8GEvmfg

Bregman, Rutger. Poverty isn't a lack of character; it's a lack of cash.
https://www.ted.com/talks/rutger_bregman_poverty_isn_t_a_lack_of_character_it_s_a_lack_of_cash

Cohen, Glenn. Are There Non-human Persons? Are There Non-person Humans? (TEDxCambridge)
https://www.youtube.com/watch?v=8Z8MMS0Su4o

Doudna, Jennifer. We can now edit our DNA but let's do it wisely
https://www.ted.com/talks/jennifer_doudna_we_can_now_edit_our_dna_but_let_s_do_it_wisely

Enriquez, Juan. We can reprogram life. How to do it wisely
https://www.ted.com/talks/juan_enriquez_we_can_reprogram_life_how_to_do_it_wisely

Fallon, James. The Moth: Confessions of a Pro-Social Psychopath (World Science Festival)
https://www.youtube.com/watch?v=fzqn6Z_Iss0

Feldman-Barrett, Lisa You aren't at the mercy of your emotions -- your brain creates them
https://www.ted.com/talks/lisa_feldman_barrett_you_aren_t_at_the_mercy_of_your_emotions_your_brain_creates_them

Film Ideas, Inc. I, psychopath
https://topdocumentaryfilms.com/i-psychopath/

Ford, Martin: How we'll earn money in a future without jobs
https://www.youtube.com/watch?v=swB7Ivct8d8

Generous, Alix. How I learned to communicate my inner life with Asperger's
http://www.ted.com/talks/alix_generous_how_i_learned_to_communicate_my_inner_life_with_asperger_s

Grandin, Temple. The world needs all kinds of minds
http://www.ted.com/talks/temple_grandin_the_world_needs_all_kinds_of_minds

Grannon. Richard. Narcissistic Abuse: An Unspoken Reality (Short Documentary)
https://youtu.be/rLCPDYt1wYk

Jegede, Faith. What I've learned from my autistic brothers
http://www.ted.com/talks/faith_jegede_what_i_ve_learned_from_my_autistic_brothers

Jorgenson, Ellen. What you need to know about CRISPR
https://www.ted.com/talks/ellen_jorgensen_what_you_need_to_know_about_crispr

Kahn, Jennifer. Gene editing can now change an entire species forever
https://www.ted.com/talks/jennifer_kahn_gene_editing_can_now_change_an_entire_species_forever

King, Rosie. How autism freed me to be myself
http://www.ted.com/talks/rosie_king_how_autism_freed_me_to_be_myself

Knoepfler, Paul. The ethical dilemma of designer babies
https://www.ted.com/talks/paul_knoepfler_the_ethical_dilemma_of_designer_babies

Lanier, Heather. "Good" and "bad" are incomplete stories we tell ourselves
https://www.ted.com/talks/heather_lanier_good_and_bad_are_incomplete_stories_we_tell_ourselves

Marsh, Abigail. Why some people are more altruistic than others.
https://www.ted.com/talks/abigail_marsh_why_some_people_are_more_altruistic_than_others/

McGonigal, Jane. Gaming can make a better world
https://www.ted.com/talks/jane_mcgonigal_gaming_can_make_a_better_world

McGonigal, Kelly. How to make stress your friend
https://www.ted.com/talks/kelly_mcgonigal_how_to_make_stress_your_friend

Noble, Kimberly. How does income affect childhood brain development?
https://www.youtube.com/watch?v=xTra-yePY_A

# Sources of information

Ockelford, Adam. Derek Paravicini and Adam Ockelford in the key of genius
http://www.ted.com/talks/derek_paravicini_and_adam_ockelford_in_the_key_of_genius

Piff, Paul. Does money make you mean?
http://www.ted.com/talks/paul_piff_does_money_make_you_mean

Pixar. "The Making of Loop" Documentary
https://www.youtube.com/watch?v=dew-zbf9BDE

Real Stories. Real Life Psychopaths (Crime Psychology Documentary)
https://www.youtube.com/watch?v=60vK6Uw9sSE

Robinson, Ken. Schools kill creativity
https://www.ted.com/talks/ken_robinson_says_schools_kill_creativity

Rosling, Hans. Let my dataset change your mindset
https://www.ted.com/talks/hans_rosling_at_state

Savulescu, Julian. The Perfect Human Being Series E01 - on human enhancement
https://www.youtube.com/watch?v=4qary81ymWk&t=993s

Saxe, Rebecca. The neuroscience of hate
https://vimeo.com/333105887

Solomon, Andrew. Love, no matter what
https://www.ted.com/talks/andrew_solomon_love_no_matter_what

Wegrzyn, Renee. Engineering Gene Safety
http://longnow.org/seminars/02017/oct/30/engineering-gene-safety/

Wilkinson, Richard. How economic inequality harms societies
http://www.ted.com/talks/richard_wilkinson

**We need to talk about this**

# About the author

According to the urban slang dictionary, she's a boss. Angelina Souren is not into consumerism, is a feminist, went to university relatively late in life and goes her own way. She's been residing in southern England since 2004, but is currently in the Netherlands. She's previously lived in balmy and blissful Florida as well as in Amsterdam and its environs. In England, she became otherized pretty badly.

She is a former board member of the Environmental Chemistry (and Toxicology) Section of the Royal Netherlands Chemical Society and a former associate editor of the international newsletter of the U.S.-based Geochemical Society. She also used to be very active in the NIMF foundation, a Dutch network for women in science and technology, which she joined in 1988 when she was still working on her Master's degree. There was only one female earth scientist among the faculty at the department from which she graduated.

Souren is a highly versatile independent critical thinker and researcher with a solid background in earth & life sciences and an interest in (bio)ethics sensu lato, hence she is also an advocate for nonhuman animals. She learned a great deal about rehabbing wild birds as a volunteer in the U.S., where she adopted two rescued wild quaker parrots who went on to teach her a heck of a lot about avians. She emigrated with them twice.

For a long time, she wanted to become a full professor with her own cutting-edge marine biogeochemistry group, preferably in the U.S. Then she discovered that it is also highly enjoyable and equally challenging as well as rewarding to be your own boss and work with an international network of associates to serve clients from a wide variety of backgrounds.

Prior to her scientific endeavors, she was employed in tourism and hospitality in Amsterdam, then decided to hand in her notice and enrolled as a full-time earth science student. Among other things, she also has several years of legal experience (English law), is a former member of Toastmasters of The Hague as well as of the Amsterdam American Business Club.

She enjoys brainstorming with highly driven smart people who set high standards for themselves. She likes the idea of creating positive change, but she knows very well that the latter is often preceded by turmoil.

**IS CRUELTY COOL?**

If you want to connect with her, you could follow her at angelinasouren.com as well as on Amazon, of course, and a few other places on the web provided it's not a Facebook-owned medium.

Liked this book? Write a review. Sorry, the t-shirt sold out pretty quickly. Disliked the book? Contact Angelina at angelinasouren@gmail.com or through her website.

www.ingramcontent.com/pod-product-compliance
Lightning Source LLC
Chambersburg PA
CBHW070636220526
45466CB00001B/187